EASY GOING

EASY GOING

A Guide to Traveling in Good Health & Good Spirits

by Mel London

 Rodale Press, Emmaus, Pa.

Printed in the United States of America on recycled paper containing a high percentage of de-inked fiber.

Book design by Ed Courrier

Library of Congress Cataloging in Publication Data

London, Mel.
  Easy going.

  Includes index.
  1. Travel. I. Title.
G151.L66   910'.2'02   80-29177
ISBN 0-87857-331-3 hardcover
ISBN 0-87857-345-3 paperback

2 4 6 8 10 9 7 5 3 1   hardcover
2 4 6 8 10 9 7 5 3 1   paperback

FOR MY FATHER, HARRY LONDON
for giving me my values for
traveling through life
and
FOR MY BROTHER, STAN
who kept me from being
an only child

Other Books by Mel London

Getting Into Film
(Ballantine Books 1977)

Bread Winners
(Rodale Press 1979)

With Sheryl London:

The Fish-Lovers' Cookbook
(Rodale Press 1980)

CONTENTS

CHAPTER 5: SITTING, RUNNING, JUMPING, STANDING, JOGGING, SLEEPING, AND BREATHING. 43

CHAPTER 6: "STOP THE SHIP—I WANT TO GET OFF!!". 59

ACKNOWLEDGMENTS

I keep rediscovering that books are not written alone. When I look at my records showing all the people who offered guidance, assistance, and information, I am always overwhelmed at the number and slightly uneasy with the feeling that, perhaps, unwittingly, I have left someone out of this list. It would be a distressing omission.

In my last two books for Rodale, I had saved my acknowledgment for my editor, Charles Gerras, for last. He has been "last but not least" too many times. This time he is first, where he belongs, and I would like to thank him once again for his encouragement and for his laughter at the stories that I was not sure were funny to anyone else but me. He has my deepest thanks and love.

The airlines and the travel organizations were all gracious and giving of their time and information. The list is long: Pan American, Japan Air Lines, Scandinavian Air Lines, Lufthansa German Airlines, and TWA. Also, Amtrak, Greyhound International, Alice Marshall of Cunard, Holland-America Cruises, the British Tourist Authority, the Port Authority of New York and New Jersey, the Department of Tourist Development for the State of Tennessee, and Victoria Foote of the French Government Tourist Office.

And there are more—so many more to whom I owe my thanks and my gratitude for their help: the American Hotel and Motel Association, the U.S. Travel Service (U.S. Department of Commerce), the U.S. Department of Agriculture, the Civil Aeronautics Board, and the Federal Aviation Administration.

In the area of health and travel, many people and organizations assisted in making the information accurate and valuable for the traveler: Dr. Eugene J.

Gangarosa, Dean of Faculty of Health Sciences, American University in Beirut; the American Foundation for the Blind; Pat McKee of the Lighthouse for the Blind; Society for Advancement of Travel for the Handicapped; Dr. Robert Dille of the Civil Aeromedical Institute, Federal Aviation Administration, in Oklahoma City; the National Institutes of Health and the Center for Disease Control of the Department of Health, Education and Welfare; New York Heart Association; Connecticut Public Health Service; the New York Diabetes Association—with a special nod to Dr. Samuel Mirsky and to the Squibb Pharmaceutical Company, for permission to use their book on traveling with diabetes.

I take a deep breath and go on: Deak-Perera as well as Manfra, Tordella & Brookes for their advice about currency, my friends at Maytag—Jan Cooper and Max Fuller—for teaching me how to do laundry while on the road, and Jane Haberern for suggesting the title of this book and encouraging me to go ahead with it.

The American Society of Travel Agents (ASTA) was invaluable to me—as was the Institute of Certified Travel Agents—and my own travel agent, Chris Miele, deserves a book of her own for what she has taught me about travel and how to enjoy it.

For this book, since Charles Gerras can no longer be "last but not least," I have saved the spot for my remarkable researcher, Deborah Goodwin, who found information where I was certain it did not exist, who collected so much of the good advice that is now included in these pages, and who kept her good humor throughout, in spite of the fact that I am not generally known as the easiest of bosses.

I do—I genuinely do—thank them all, each and every one, and may they find all their trips "Easy Going."

Mel London
Fire Island, New York

INTRODUCTION

My mother was my first travel agent. Even if the trip was up the street to Eli's candy store, I was prepared and dressed and armed with enough information to have sent Stanley off to find Livingston. "Don't go out with a wet head!" It was the first bit of travel/health advice that I can remember. It still haunts me when I leave a hotel room in some far-off place like Nairobi, having just taken a shower. The echo of her voice rings in my ear: "Wait until your hair dries before you go out!"

"Pin your mittens to your mackinaw" and "Let someone take you across the street" were other homilies that passed as travel advice, though it became a bit embarrassing when I was old enough to join the Boy Scouts and my mother made me promise to ask old ladies to watch *me* cross the street while on my way to the troop meetings. She never got over it. When I left to enlist in the army, my mother watched out of our third-story Bronx apartment window to see that no cars were speeding down the hill.

Of course, it has been a lot of years since then, and over two million miles have passed beneath the airplanes and the ships and the cars I've ridden. As a destination, Eli's candy store has given way to more than 60 countries around the world. Now my travel agent is a professional who gives other good advice. As a filmmaker, I travel 150,000 miles in a slow year, while in the year just passed, it has probably been closer to 250,000 miles.

To complicate matters, each trip changes character, and a new set of problems arises with every schedule, with every project. There are times when my crew and I are based in Paris or Rome or some other exquisite oasis of civilization. More often than not, though, the job takes us to one of the world's more colorful slums or to the backwater villages of a developing South American country. I love it. I have always loved it, and I guess I will always find myself lying awake the night before a trip, anticipating the new adventure, the new people, the excitement, even the trials and tribulations. It even happens to me when I am about to leave for Detroit or Cleveland the next morning. I am a hopeless and inveterate travel "junkie," and it will always be so.

Travel has not been without its problems. Our crews change often—three to five people with different personalities, different needs, and different health problems. Above all, though, there is a pragmatic need to accomplish the job efficiently, to keep on schedule, and to keep everyone healthy enough to function in some of the worst areas that the world has to offer. In our travels, if we lose a day through illness, through a crew member contracting Montezuma's Revenge or the Tourist Trots (or whatever it's called in that particular part of the world), the financial burden becomes a problem, schedules are backed up, and our production timetable suffers as much as our spirits. In an Asian city where there are only two flights a week to the outside world, even one day of illness can be a major catastrophe.

It is remarkable that, in these wonderful 35 years of traveling the globe, my crews have rarely been sick and I have been ill only four times—twice in South America and twice in one of America's leading fast-food chains. I have since discovered the problem in South America (meat that was not cooked thoroughly enough), but I have not chanced going back to Ptomaine Emporium to find out what went wrong.

Naturally, we all like to give advice, and through these years, I have given freely of my wisdom to friends who are about to embark on trips of their own. Often my counsel is ignored. After all, none of us likes exactly the same things, few of us are built the same, and most of us are susceptible to different viruses. My film partner of 16 years drinks water from any tap in the world, eats anything that is put in front of him, and claims that he has never been sick a day in his travel life. He also claims that all illness is psychosomatic, and I, in turn, have told him that this book is not for him!

For my other friends who have ignored my good advice over all these years, I have decided to write *Easy Going*, for the printed word is often more authoritative and threatening than the ramblings of a jaded traveler given freely over the table at a dinner party. For those of you who will listen, I want to share my joy of travel with you, my adventures, my excitement about the world. At the same time, I want to give you some armament to make your trips memorable and safe enough to have you return and regale *me* with your own experiences. I would even be willing to sit through your out-of-focus slide shows of the marketplace in Chichicastenango.

To be realistic, though, many of my friends return with tales of illness, especially on their trips to the more out-of-the-way places in this world. It's unfortunate, for I firmly believe that good health on a trip goes hand in hand with having a good time. A few rules of common sense, and the journey can become an easy one. I read an article recently in which a tour guide complained that her group would not listen to her advice about the food and water, and all had become violently ill on the very first day. Ironically, the group consisted of 40 doctors and their spouses!

I do not mean to imply that no useful travel books exist anywhere else. The shelves are crowded with colorful temptations that seduce us with the tropical coral reefs of the South Pacific, but they fail to include any warning about the danger of walking on those reefs. The pamphlets issued by local governments and tourist offices make bewitching promises of golden temples and nights under the full moon, but, understandably enough, they don't mention the fact that the local water supply is the equivalent of cyanide for visitors. An occasional article in the newspaper comments on jet lag or motion sickness. Pamphlets are available from government agencies about health and immunization, and there have even been several books devoted specifically to the health problems you meet around the world.

In *Easy Going,* I have put down on paper some of my own thoughts about what is important in travel. These suggestions reflect my personal experience and discoveries as well as the recommendations of experts.

I am tired of seeing inexperienced travelers being taken advantage of by airlines, tour guides, and hotels around the world. And so I have added some words about travelers' rights. Friends of mine, in turn, have given me their own good tips about their wanderings, and I pass them on to you. So, in the pages that follow, you will also find words about laundry, customs declarations and problems, currency and tipping, as well as some language stories that may help you get past the first few days in a strange and distant land.

This book, to put it simply, is my personal potpourri of information about the world, based upon 35 years of wandering through it. It tells about how best to survive in it, while having that same world give you the fullest nourishment that it has to offer. If we let it envelop us, if we remain flexible enough to devour its wonders, intelligent enough to meet its challenges, then every journey we take, no matter how close to home or how far away, will be worth our while.

When you have finished reading this book, you may choose, as some of my friends have, to strike off on your own in your own way, depending upon your own common sense, not mine, and upon the advice of your own personal friends, not mine. It matters not. I only ask that, as you begin your journey, you remember but two firm bits of advice:

- Look both ways before crossing the street (especially where they drive on the left-hand side)!

- Don't go out with a wet head!

"GOODBYE AND HELLO"

The Time Before Leaving . . . Travel Books . . .
Tickets, Passports, and Other
Interesting Documents . . .

A nontraveler friend of mine used to expound on his theories of staying at home by saying, "I don't want to go anyplace I haven't been, I don't want to meet anybody I haven't met, and I don't want to taste anything I haven't eaten before!" For him, and for others like him, the world is a foreign place filled with foreign devils, where there is no doubt that the food and water will make him violently ill, where the souvenirs will be horrendously overpriced, the hotel rooms crawling with vermin, the language a cross between Polish spoken backwards and hieroglyphics—and, frankly, if that's the way he sees it, that's the way it will be. Keep in mind, however, that his attitude need not be applied only to the underdeveloped areas of the world. Many people feel exactly the same way about visiting my own home city, New York! Fortunately, my friend does not travel much.

There are others who do leave home and then return to state rather imperiously, "We had a marvelous trip. We didn't go to any of the places that the tourists visit!" The word *tourists* is generally accompanied by a sneer. Projecting their trip in my own mind, I assume that if they just came back

1

from Paris, then they missed the Louvre, the Eiffel Tower, the Left Bank, and Notre Dame. If they were in North Africa, the Casbah was untouched, and Hong Kong was overlooked entirely on their jaunt through Hong Kong.

IT ALL ADDS UP
TO ATTITUDE

What I am trying to say is that a sense of the right *attitude* is probably the best preparation that anyone can give to another traveler. Some years ago it was considered a fact, for example, that all of us Americans were loved wherever we went. It was never true, but we liked to *believe* it was. We were, after all, Americans, and nothing could happen to us. What a rude awakening when we found that our young people could be—and were being—arrested and jailed for carrying drugs across the border of Turkey, or that some hostile crowds were hostile *only* because we were Americans.

I remember my years of travel through South America and the difference in our reception depending upon something as simple as who was the president at that particular moment. During the time of Nixon, we were treated with hostility and disdain, in sharp contrast to the greetings and the governmental assistance we received while John Kennedy was in the White House. During the years of the anti-Vietnam demonstrations in Sydney, Australia, our entire group donned Canadian lapel flags in order to walk the streets loved and unscathed.

And so I begin a book called *Easy Going* with stories of hostility and mobs shouting outside the embassies, and my nontraveling friend seizes the opportunity to say, "See? I told you so!" Yet I found it exciting, and I still do. And when someone asks me what I did through all that turmoil, I answer, "I smiled a lot!" (And kept my fingers crossed.) For such experiences comprise but a small percentage of the two million miles and the 35 years. And they do, indeed, make good storytelling when you get home. The other 99 percent of the time, we opened ourselves to what the world had to show us and we grew from it and became more understanding of just who makes up the rest of the human race. Certainly, it is easier to stay at home than to remove ourselves from a familiar environment, particularly if the final destination is foreign to our cultural background. But, for many of us—and I include anyone who would even pick up a travel book to read it—the challenge whets the appetite even more. The next trip cannot come too soon.

BEFORE DEPARTURE

I believe that there are two major attributes that a traveler needs. The first is flexibility, and it will stand you in good stead no matter where you are, no matter what situation befalls you. The second is an ability to plan well. The trip begins long before you drive to the airport or to the steamship terminal. If papers are in order, if health and prevention rules are followed, if everything is taken care of at home, if you know as much as possible about your destinations, you will probably have fewer unexpected things befall you during your trip. Now notice that I did not promise *nothing* would befall you, and I did insert the word *probably*. The qualifications only promise *fewer* unexpected disasters. After all, part of the beauty of travel is surprise and discovery—which brings us back to the first attribute that I mentioned: flexibility!

For many of us, the planning of the trip is part of the fun, as it should be. And the rules are still the same whether or not you use a travel agent in conjunction with that planning. (In Chapter 2, I will cover the role of the travel agent and give you some tips on how to choose one.) Begin by getting all the information you possibly can about the places you're going to visit.

TRANSLATE TRAVEL
TIPS FROM FRIENDS

Part of the information—or misinformation—will, of course, come from friends who have already been there. This advice can be valuable to a first-time visitor, but keep in mind that we all like different things, that a "charming" hotel to them might well be a "rat trap" to you. Probably, you have never traveled with them. Your relationship is close, but it revolves around your hometown social amenities and dinners together at the same restaurants; your time together probably does not exceed a few hours a week or a month. Have you ever *lived* with them for two weeks or a month, shared with them their openness or hostility to something new or different?

I remember thinking that I knew some people rather well. We had seen them for years as close acquaintances here in the United States. By accident, we ran into them in Kyoto, Japan, and they asked us to their room. Now I am a very neat traveler. Everything has a place in my temporary "home" for the night. I pride myself on being able to get in and out of a hotel in ten minutes at the most. And so, when they opened their door, a new view, a new discovery struck me. Apparently, the room had been hit by a typhoon! Clothes were strewn around the beds, the dressers, the chairs. Underwear hung from the light fixture; suitcases were open, and clothing dripped from the sides onto the floor. It was a part of them I had never known. I swore then that I would never travel with them—ever.

I have found that most film crew members are flexible, charming, efficient, helpful, and open—while in the United States. Suddenly, on the first overseas trip, Dr. Jekyll turns into Mr. Hyde. Twice during my film career, I have fired people while we were overseas and sent them home. So remember that you are your own person, and, though you can get plenty of good advice from your friends, your own investigation, your own search, your own quest for knowledge will be far more valuable to you on your trip. (And here you are taking advice from the author, a perfect stranger!)

GUIDEBOOKS, BROCHURES, AND OTHER CREATIVE WRITING

There are, of course, the guidebooks. They're good places to begin. They do have a tendency to glorify things, of course, but they can be excellent sources of information about hotels, currency, tipping, electrical currents, places to visit, local customs, festivals, and the other information that you need to give you the flavor of a country. Just make certain that you read the latest guide available, for the same information about the Tower of London may be there through every edition of the book, but hotels, restaurants, currency values, and even connecting roads change from year to year.

OFFICIAL TOURIST OFFICES

The tourist offices are also good places to get brochures, maps, and travel information, as is the consulate of the country to which you're traveling. If the trip is domestic, write to the chamber of commerce of the city or state, or to the national park or the resort or hotel that you've chosen. Again, with all of these, keep in mind that the photographs and descriptive material will always be positive (which they should be). But the photograph of the young, gorgeous couple lying suntanned and oiled on the beach may not be typical of the tropical paradise to which you are flying. You will never see the beautiful couple. In fact, there may not even be a beach!

TRAVEL DOCUMENTS

Make certain you find out about the travel documents and the immunizations required for travel to a particular destination, about currency exchange, about the weather, and about the clothing you'll need. Check into the local shopping bargains. Frequently, you can get the same things cheaper at home. We may not like to think so, but it's true more often than we care to admit.

Today, bookstores carry a large display of travel books. It seems that nearly everyone goes somewhere on vacation or on business, and even our smaller cities are catering to that new wanderlust. However, if your local bookstore doesn't have what you specifically want or need, try writing to a little shop that I've discovered in New York. It has a remarkable collection of travel material, from guides to maps, from dictionaries to currency converters. It's called The Complete Traveler and is located at 199 Madison Avenue, New York, NY 10016 (telephone: 212-679-4339).

Years ago, when we spoke of "areas of unrest," we usually meant a country or a continent that had seldom even seen a tourist. Today, the world has changed, and our daily newspapers tell us that one day's tropical paradise is another day's arena of revolution. If you're a business traveler or a tourist who is going to an area that might be uncertain or volatile, you would do well to carry with you a booklet called *Key Offices of Foreign Service Posts.* It lists the United States missions abroad, and it can be obtained from the U.S. Government Printing Office, Washington, DC 20402 ($1.50). Certainly, there is no guarantee that the telephones listed will even be working when you get to the area, and, even if they are, the consul or the mission staff may be of little help, but I carry the booklet anyhow. It's a link, someone to turn to.

THE FLEXIBLE
AIRLINE TICKET

If you're not using a travel agent, it's good to check the airline fares and regulations rather thoroughly. As a traveling businessman, I have found that I am eligible for very few of the special rates offered by the carriers. My trips are generally too short or too long, or they are not planned far enough in advance, or they have the wrong stopovers. But most people do have the time. It just takes a bit of effort to find out what is available, and the savings can be substantial. At one time, it was a fairly simple matter to make the choice, but since the deregulation of the airlines, it has become more and more complicated. New, small carriers have entered and expanded service on the routes formerly served by only a few. Day and night rates vary considerably. Frills (for whatever they were worth) have been removed from some routes, with a resultant lowering of fares.

The time of year that you travel is important, and only a few days' change in plans might well move you into "off season" rates. The airlines have offered all kinds of money-saving promotions, from discount coupons to half-fares, for only limited periods of time. These are particularly prevalent when an airline enters a new route. Watch for them.

The Civil Aeronautics Board, in its excellent little pamphlet *Fly Rights* (Civil Aeronautics Board, Washington, DC 20428), sums up the tips rather well. Keep in mind that these are for flying within the United States. The guidelines for foreign carriers are just about the same, however, even though their fares are set by the International Air Transport Association (IATA).

• Call or write the individual airline and ask for a summary of routes and fares. If you're in a larger city, a visit to the individual airline office will help. But remember that each airline is out to sell its own schedule rather than that of its competitor.

• Try to be as flexible as possible in your travel plans. Many times there are complex conditions that you'll have to meet in order to qualify for lower fares—departure on specific days, minimum length of stay, limited stopovers, and so forth. We have found, at times, that by adding an extra stop or by eliminating one, a fare may drop drastically. This is particularly true for overseas travel.

• Try to plan your itinerary as far ahead as you possibly can. The budget seats on a plane are limited, and it's first come, first served until they're gone.

• It's important that you find out just what happens to your fare if you switch flights or change the date of departure. In some instances, you lose the discount; in others, the airline levies a stiff penalty for cancelling or changing your plans.

• Get your ticket early. Once you have your ticket, you will not be liable for any fare increase. However, if you merely have a confirmed reservation, when you pick up your ticket you'll have to pay any intervening overcharges. With the escalating cost of jet fuel, the conditions seem to change daily.

Incidentally, cruise lines have been offering an interesting way to save on fares. Though the dollar value of the ticket has remained fairly constant over these past few years, the cruises have merely been *shortened* by several days to meet rising costs. Unfortunately, the airlines cannot follow suit—a ten-hour trip remains a ten-hour trip.

OTHER TICKETS, OTHER SAVINGS

We poor, downtrodden business people are usually not able to take advantage of travel bargains. As a part of your planning, check the tourist office or consulate of the country you are about to visit, specifically to find out if they offer discount passes for tourists. For many years, some countries allowed travelers with rental cars to discount their gas purchases. Even then, with a gallon of fuel at nearly two dollars, it was a bargain that was hard to resist. For the most part, it is a "perk" that is long gone, as gas prices go higher and higher.

There are still some governments that issue rail and tourist discount passes, but remember that they must be purchased *before* you leave the United States. The most popular of these is the well-known Eurailpass, which allows you unlimited first-class train travel in 15 European countries, with a time limit of from 15 days to three months. In a few instances, the pass also includes some travel on inland waterways and lakes. (The pass excludes Great Britain, by the way.)

There is another advantage to the passes these days. The dollar keeps fluctuating, which is a polite word for saying that in many places it just isn't worth what it used to be. Be prepared for escalating prices in most countries in the world. A pass purchased far in advance is immune to any price changes after you arrive.

British Rail also has a pass available for tourists, as do Germany, Denmark, Norway, Finland, Sweden, and Italy. France offers an unlimited air pass, while many countries, including Britain and Italy, sell passes that give you huge discounts for museums, castles, and historical sites.

It is important to check into these possibilities when you're planning your trip. Ask the tourist offices, question the airlines, read the travel ads in your local newspaper. The offers change, and any list of them here would soon be out of date. For example, at the time of this writing, Portugal is offering a free night at a hotel as a part of its travel bargain, but this could change tomorrow. The tourist industry is always competing for the travel dollar, and the smart shopper knows how to take advantage of it.

"MY,
WHAT A BEAUTIFUL
PASSPORT PHOTO!"

The phrase above has probably never been uttered. It is my personal opinion that passport photographers go to "ugly" school just to learn "flat" lighting, get the wrong expression on the subject's face, and do it all in 30 seconds. It sometimes amazes me that Customs Officers in foreign countries can actually recognize that the photo in my passport is really a likeness of me!

Nevertheless, when you have the photos taken, even though they're ugly, get about ten extra copies. You may not think you need any others, but many visa applications still require passport photos to be attached. In addition, international driver's licenses also require them, and there are even ski lodges that attach your picture to the lift pass. I always carry an envelope with about ten photos in it, and I keep it at the bottom of my travel bag. It has come in handy. Too, if you should have the god-awful experience of having your passport lost or stolen, the extra photos will expedite issuance of a new passport by the nearest American consulate.

SOME TIPS
ON SECURITY

Before taking off on your trip:

• Make note of your passport number and carry it separately.

• Tell one of your neighbors just where you'll be and how to get in touch with you. Leave a copy of your itinerary.

• Photocopy all your credit cards and any other papers you might have to take with you. Take one copy along and leave the other with your neighbor or with someone who is staying at home.

• Do the same with your traveler's checks (more about that in Chapter 23, on currency and tipping). Make a list of their numbers and leave it at home; carry a duplicate list with you—*but not with the checks themselves,* or, if the checks are stolen, your list will be gone too.

• If you are taking any foreign-made equipment with you—cameras, computers, tape recorders—have it registered with U.S. Customs before you leave, so that you will not have to prove that it was purchased here and is not subject to duty. This can be done at the international airport, but be sure to allow enough time, and—if you are departing at 3:00 A.M.— telephone first to make sure that a Customs Officer is, indeed, on duty at that hour. If you're carrying expensive jewelry, take your insurance appraisal form with you.

• Cancel all mail and newspaper service to your home if it is to be unattended. Also cancel any other deliveries that might indicate that you are not at home, such as laundry or milk service.

• If your town is a small one, ask the local police to check your home from time to time. We find that we can do this in our small community on Fire Island, but it becomes more complex—in fact, impossible—in New York City.

• Some travel guides recommend that you set timers and lights to go on and off at certain hours. I have never been sold on the theory, ever since I read somewhere that some thieves like to *look* for lights that go on and off at certain times and then enter the house. It is less suspicious, they said, for someone to see a figure in a lighted house than to spot the beam of a flashlight flickering around a room. I leave the decision up to you.

Though this chapter seems to be devoted to overseas travel, most of what has been said can apply to domestic travel as well. Certainly, you won't need a passport to visit Los Angeles or Miami, but there *are* discounts available, the airlines sometimes offer free hotels or coupon books for restaurants and amusement parks, and the rules about currency, traveler's checks, and locking your house should apply for any trip.

AND BEFORE
YOU LEAVE

There is one final thing that guarantees that you have done all you possibly could before your departure. Walk through your trip in your head. Start from the beginning—check the airline tickets, mentally arrive at each hotel, check the dates and the travel connections. In our film business, the production managers go through exactly that process before they send a crew on the road. You'd be surprised how many times they discover an error (usually blamed on a computer).

In spite of all this, of course, things will happen. You're probably asking right now just what misbegotten circumstances the author has gotten into over these long years. The answer is, "Plenty!" With all of our checking and double-checking, with all of our planning, there are still things that go wrong, cars that are not there to meet us, accidents, cancelled flights, nonexistent guaranteed (doubly) hotel rooms, and, inevitably, those damned computers. Sometimes, however, the problem is a human one.

We had planned our trip to a small dictatorship in Asia with great care. Getting film equipment in and out was difficult enough, and getting permission to film was even more complex. The colonels, put in by the "strong man," just didn't want us there. Tourists, yes; film crews, no. I made a long, tiring trip to the country just to meet with the colonels—22 hours in the air, and I was virtually prostrate with jet lag. We talked for most of a day, and finally they agreed to let us enter the country in two months' time. I went back to my people tired but overjoyed.

Two months later, everything else having been checked for the hundredth time, our crew of six took off and arrived at 1:00 A.M. (after a flight of the same 22 hours), and we found the country still under heavy martial law. Perversely, it was good to be back, even with the armed soldiers patrolling the airport. A messenger came up to me—I was to report to the colonels at 10:00 A.M. "After the long flight? We had planned to sleep." "Yes, sir. There seems to be some doubt about your shooting permit."

At 10:00 A.M. I arrived, my head filled with the buzzing of gnats, my eyes at half-mast, my mouth tasting of the Japanese noodles we had eaten all the way across the Pacific. The smile that I wore as I entered the room soon dropped into an unbelieving frown. The colonels were there, all right, but they seemed to be the *wrong* colonels. The strong man had replaced every single one of the people I had previously met, *all* the colonels were different. Why, they wanted to know, did I want to film in their country? This was no survey trip. If they refused permission now, the entire trip was wasted, the losses astronomical to fly six people to Asia and then home again without shooting one foot of film. Somehow, it worked out. Somehow, in my jet-lag-filled brain, I came up with the answers that satisfied them all. It took four hours, but again we got permission to shoot. In fact, the colonels and I ended up discussing the production of an eventual tourist film in their dictatorship!

Such is the serendipity of travel!

2

HOW TO FALL IN LOVE WITH YOUR TRAVEL AGENT

... Or Merely to Choose a Good One

In my early days of travel, I did it all alone. My first world trip in 1961 taught me how to select airlines; choose hotels; read the schedules in the *Official Airline Guide;* select overland transportation; enter mortal combat with recalcitrant agents, hotel clerks, and tour guides; find electricity where none was listed in the books; have my laundry done; avoid the water, the ice, the food, the heat, the cold, and the altitude; dress properly; wear the right shoes; take care of skin rashes, snakebite, and fevers—and then, 20 years later, wonder how I was able to do it all. I would not do it again. I just did not know enough to let someone else take the responsibility.

TO USE OR NOT TO USE AN AGENT

I wish I could say that I then found a wonderful travel agent who let me relax and who took everything off my delicate and overworked hands.

Unfortunately, I did not. My first travel agents just did not understand me or my problems. At least, that's what I thought. It may well have been my own handicap in not being able to communicate my specific needs to them. But finding a good agent took years and many trips; it took a series of situations in which I stood stranded in some foreign desert with the wrong airline ticket in my hand, even though I thought I had checked everything before leaving the United States.

Finding a travel agent is like looking for a doctor. It's totally emotional, and you must have an empathy with the agent who is sending you off on your trip. At the beginning, you'll have no idea whether you're getting good or bad advice, but if the confidence is there and your agent turns out to be a good one, the relationship can be worth your sanity. My own story has a happy ending. About ten years ago, our company found a travel agent who combined all the patience, good humor, expertise, knowledge, and instinct that makes for a good travel manager. Her name is Chris Miele, and, considering the difficulties that arise in handling film crews (changed schedules, rewritten tickets, last-minute emergencies), she is certain to be nominated as a saint.

I must add that I am glad I had the experience of planning all my own trips for so many years. It helps tremendously when we are far from home and some changes must be made because the monsoon has destroyed our shooting schedule or a hotel doesn't have the "guaranteed" reservation. But with a good travel agent now, I feel that I have Utopia.

HOW TRAVEL AGENTS WORK

One thing should be understood before beginning any discussion about travel agents, however: The service is free to the customer. The agents' pay is the commission they get from the airlines, hotels, car rental agencies, steamship lines, guide services, and all the other areas that go to make up your trip. The inexperienced traveler's first reaction, then, is that agents probably try to book you on the most expensive routes possible, put you up in the King Tut suite, and feed you three-star French gourmet dinners in order to keep their commissions high. This is just not true with a good agent. I have seen Chris spend hours with the computers and on the telephone to find another way to route our crews, in order to save us some money. Remember that the travel agent is a business person, and your repeat trips as well as your recommendations can mean the difference between failure and success, especially if their business is a small, local one.

13

TYPES OF
TRAVEL AGENCIES

There are basically two types of travel agencies:

• The ticket agency, one that takes only reservations for travel and issues tickets for the trip.

• The full-service travel agency, handling everything you can think of to make the trip complete—hotels, airlines, cruise ships, railroads, car rentals, guided tours, tips on clothing, climate, luggage, visas, passports, local conditions, and even guidance on local shopping and bargain hunting.

WHAT THE AGENT
CAN DO FOR YOU

It is quite possible that my early experiences with travel agents also had a built-in problem of which I was unaware. In those early days, I guess I had been traveling to places that my agent had not visited. I knew (or thought I knew) more about the hotels and food and airline connections in Pakistan than the agent did. For the most part, this is no longer true. Most travel agents have become world travelers themselves. My own agent has visited almost every destination to which we have reason to travel. That, combined with the stories told by returning customers and the study of industry reports and literature, makes today's agent quite knowledgeable about the world in which we live. Also, the airlines and steamship lines often run "junkets" for agents, in order to introduce them to services, new routes, hotels, and tour availabilities. Though, unlike you and me, agents are treated like royalty on these junkets, the experience does help them to understand more about their clients' travel problems.

From a very pragmatic point of view, agents have much more "clout" than we do, in many areas. They provide such a huge volume of business for the travel industry that they frequently can open space for accommodations where none seems to be available. The carriers and the hotels will deny it vehemently, but many do hold space available for their best customers, namely the agents.

With the new computer systems that are being installed all over the country, many of them right in the office of the travel agent, today's rapidly

14

changing airline schedules are available and accurate up to the minute when you call or come into the office. American Airlines with its 1700 SABRE computers, TWA and its PARS system, United with its APOLLO, and ITT with its multiaccess computer terminals have made it a joy to telephone our agent and get a confirmation right on the spot. By the push of a button, the ticket can be issued automatically, or the information can be stored for future use. Of course, this doesn't mean that no mistakes are made. Certainly there are, and certainly there will be, so long as human beings and computers exist in trial marriage. But overall, knowing immediately that a flight is overbooked, that space is or is not available, that a hotel has a convention that week is a delightful change from sitting on the telephone for hours, sending expensive cables overseas, and waiting breathlessly for weeks to find out if the trip is, after all, going to happen.

DOING
YOUR HOMEWORK

There is, on the other hand, a firm responsibility on *your* part if you decide to use a travel agent. Much of the preplanning that I spoke of in Chapter 1 must still be done by you. The agent cannot read your mind (even though I am convinced that our own agent can read mine after all these years).

- You must be prepared to say just what it is you want, rather than to ask the agent what he or she can do for you. What are your preferences in hotels, sports, activities, food? You should, in fact, have a pretty clear idea as to destination, even in general terms.

- What are your budget parameters? What time limits do you have on your trip?

- What costs would you like to have included in the "package" you finally choose? What about charges levied if you cancel or if you change your reservation? Are you prepared to pay? What about charter flights — are you up on the rules governing them?

Earlier, I spoke of the colorful travel brochures. Every agent has thousands of them, and almost all of them can explain to you just what it is the trip will, or will not, include. In other words, the agent is the person best able to help you "read between the lines," so that you will not be disappointed on arrival to find out that your "luxury suite" is actually a small closet over the kitchen.

And, in planning ahead, make sure that you see your agent far enough in advance to take advantage of not only the travel bargains but also the solutions to problems of in-season travel. Incidentally, though these normal services are free, as I mentioned before, the agent does charge for unusual expenses, such as overseas cables to hotels. The earlier you book your trip, the less likely you'll have these added fees.

SOME ADVANTAGES
OF USING A
TRAVEL AGENT

There is another psychological area of "clout" that comes with using a travel agent. Though using these experts does not guarantee that you will travel problem-free, overseas and domestic hotels, car rental agencies, and sight-seeing organizations are fairly sensitive to the fact that your travel agent is necessary to their continued business. You will, of course, meet individual agents, clerks, and executives on your trip who just don't give a damn—try a crowded airline terminal during weather delay conditions, for example—but overall, there is a little more respect given to a person on an agent-booked trip than to the lonely individual who has booked it himself.

Recently, for example, we had planned a week's vacation in a South American country that was close to one in which we were to be filming. During the production, the "vacation country" had a small revolution, and we decided to cancel our rest and recuperation trip. Though telephone calls to the local travel agency in that country assured us that "everything is really all right" for tourists, returning travelers brought tales of incidents that were fairly ugly. We cancelled. Unfortunately, we had paid a rather large amount of money in advance, and, on our return, we discussed this with our agent. She was able to get a refund of everything but a small token amount for cables and a prepaid hotel. Somehow, I doubt that I could have done that alone.

Generally, then, I do recommend that you find a good agent, someone who understands you and who is sympathetic to your needs and to your budget. But when you find that special person, don't abuse the relationship. There's only so much your agent can do—or should be expected to do. You may not fall in love with your travel agent, as we have, but chances are that you'll get to like him or her an awful lot.

If you'd like further information about the services of the travel agent, here are two more sources you can pursue:

- Write to the American Society of Travel Agents (ASTA), 711 Fifth Avenue, New York, NY 10022.

- There is an excellent little paperback book called *Your Travel Agent—A Consumer's Guide* published by Dorison House, 802 Park Square Building, Boston, MA 02116 (1979, $1.95). The book is sponsored by Americana Hotels, but I found it fairly objective in its information.

3

AN OUNCE OF PREVENTION

A Dedication to Your Doctor, Your Dentist . . .
with Some Words About Immunizations

Though I suppose my vaguest, earliest memories about inoculation go back to elementary school days and some distant feeling that I must have been immunized against smallpox as a child, I cannot really remember much about it. Our generation also predated polio vaccines, and so the most vivid recollections about "shots" are the ones from my army service in what I possessively call "my war"—World War II and its vast mobilization.

It was exactly as subsequent Hollywood films would depict it, and I assure my younger readers that we did, indeed, line up, all the millions of us, naked and shivering. We didn't know whether to cover ourselves with our hands as we stood in line, or to strike a cavalier attitude telling the world that we were not really affected at all by the sight of two burly medics brandishing wicked-looking needles that looked larger and larger as we came closer to the point of no return.

Simultaneously, each medic grabbed an arm, and, in a flashing instant, it was over—I cannot even recall now what it was they were injecting: typhoid?

tetanus? In fact, we never asked! Sometimes the upper arm hurt at once. Other times, the response came later in the day through swelling, fever, and a deep ache. Some of us walked off wondering why there was so much fuss. Some, in turn, took two short steps following the shots and then fainted dead away. Things have changed.

We still get our vaccinations for the same reasons, though some diseases have almost disappeared, while others have made themselves known through our expansion of travel to more isolated parts of the world. Tour groups and individual travelers can now explore the outer limits of civilization as the globe shrinks. We think nothing of a trip to the Galápagos or Machu Picchu or Botswana. But, along with our new sense of adventure, we have also begun to hear new words like plague and dengue fever.

This, along with all the old, valid reasons for seeing a doctor before leaving on a trip, makes it even more imperative that we understand that the preventive medicine aspects of travel begin long before we embark on the plane or train or ship. We never seem to allow enough time for our well-being. We plan for months with our friends, our travel agents, our business associates, and we leave too little time to equip ourselves properly for traveling in the best of health. Yet the omission of a simple protective procedure can ruin all the plans we've made. At the very least, there are many countries that will not even allow you entry without the proper immunization. At the worst, your health can be affected for a long time after you've returned from your trip.

I am not pointing a finger. We are all guilty, and, at times, I certainly have been as flagrantly culpable as anyone. I remember a trip that we took many years back—it was to cover 15 countries, and we were to be gone for three months. Needless to say, the rush, the details, the Customs planning, the visas, letter writing, hotel arrangements kept us busy day and night. The trip to the doctor was delayed too long. One series of shots consisted of three inoculations, one week apart. We had waited so long that we could only take two of the shots, and the third would have to be given in Australia. Our doctor gave us the vaccine for the third inoculation, and, for three days, we kept it refrigerated wherever we went, even on the airplane. It became an obsession to make sure the vaccine was kept safely, for, after all, *we* were the patients for whom it was intended. We arrived in Australia, tired but happy. While going through Customs, the vaccine was confiscated by an officer who smiled icily and said, "There was no need to bring it all the way to Australia. We have the same vaccine here. We *are* civilized, you know!"

YOUR DOCTOR, YOUR DENTIST, YOUR OPTOMETRIST

But it is not only the vaccination phases of your journey that should take you to your doctor and your dentist at an early date. It makes good sense, whether you are on a trip to a neighboring state or on your way to the South Pacific. A toothache in the wrong place is enough to wreck the journey. In addition, dentistry in some parts of the world is not the most efficient science, to say the least.

Some of us wear eyeglasses—I cannot see the small print on my passport without them. Not only should you pack an extra pair of glasses in case you lose the pair you're carrying, but it's a good idea to get your prescription from your optometrist and carry it along with you in your wallet or purse.

On a trip to Asia, I had the misfortune (I really mean "stupidity") to lose my glasses in Hong Kong. Fortunately, there are optical experts every hundred feet on Nathan Road in Kowloon. While I had my lunch, new glasses were made from my prescription. I still wear them, and my own optometrist has complimented the work of the Chinese Optical Company.

If you are taking special prescription medicines, be certain that your doctor gives you enough to last the trip, plus a written prescription you can take along, just in case you run out along the way. And another good tip here is to get that prescription with the *generic* name for the drug. Many times, the medicine you're taking in the United States or Canada is merely the brand name given to it by a specific pharmaceutical company. Miltown, for example, is the manufacturer's trade name for meprobamate. Aspirin, on the other hand, is always aspirin.

YOUR MEDICAL RECORD

If you have a special problem over and above the usual ills to which we are all heir, it's also a good idea to have your doctor fill out a medical record. In Chapter 12, I will cover the specific needs of the traveler who is diabetic or who has arthritis or who travels in a wheelchair, but the preplanning for everyone should include a physical checkup at your family doctor's office. A written record should be part of your luggage if you feel that you may need special help or assistance at any time during the trip. The record can be a simple one that

Patient Identification

| | | | | | Photograph |

Surname | Given or Christian names | Birthdate
day   mo.   year

Address | Zip or postal code

Area code   phone number
(   ) | Sex (MF) | Height | Weight | Color of hair | Color of eyes | Marital status

Social insurance number | Hospital insurance number | Citizenship | Religion

In emergency notify | Relationship | Area code   phone number
(   )

Address

Emergency Medical Data

Diagnosis:

Current medication:

Antibiotic and drug sensitivities:

Allergies:

Steroid therapy in last 12 months:

Blood Type:_____ RH Factor:_____ Contact lenses:_____

Prescription for Glasses

	SPH	CYL	AXIS	PRISM	BASE
FAR R					
FAR L					
NEAR R					
NEAR L					

Signature: _____
(Oculist or Optometrist)

Diagnostic Summary

(If your patient has a cardiac condition enclose
copy of ECG. If he underwent major
surgery describe pathological findings.)

Attending physician:_____

Address:_____

_____ Phone: (   )_____

Clinical (medical) record

gives just a few items of information to another physician or hospital, such as blood type, allergies, or medication needs; or it can be much more complex and detailed. The accompanying example is a form provided by IAMAT (International Association for Medical Assistance to Travelers). I will discuss IAMAT in further detail in Chapter 20, along with a similar organization called Intermedic. Notice that IAMAT even provides warning cards for diabetics who are taking insulin, patients on anticoagulant drugs, and those of us who are susceptible to allergies.

MEDICAL BRACELETS

If you have special problems, or if you just want to be certain that you are well prepared, you may want to go a step further in providing information for

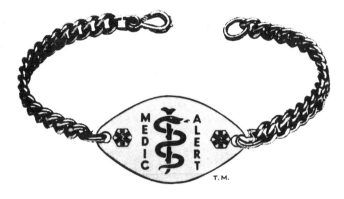

Medic Alert bracelet (physical problem identified on the underside)

emergencies. Most drugstores carry a simple medical identification bracelet on which you can detail your personal information.

However, for even more security, there is a nonprofit foundation called Medic Alert (P.O. Box 1009, Turlock, CA 95380) that registers the traveler for one small, tax-deductible, lifetime fee. You are given a personal registration number, and your medical file is recorded at Medic Alert. A bracelet or disc is then given to you, and it carries your serial number, the 24-hour (collect) telephone number of Medic Alert, and the specific problems of the wearer, such as "Taking Anticoagulants," "Allergic to Bee Stings," "Wearing Contact Lenses," "Allergic to Penicillin." Other allergies or problems can, of course, be engraved—implanted pacemaker, epilepsy, heart condition, and so on. Medic Alert has become so well known that its insignia is recognized almost everywhere, even in many countries overseas. Of course, in some areas, it may be impossible to have someone telephone Turlock, California, and, thus, I have covered other serious medical emergencies in Chapter 20.

There are also companies that will microfilm your medical history and place it in a capsule that can be worn around the neck. It has a lens at one end and microfilm at the other. By holding the lens up to the light, the profile can be read in an instant by the emergency staff. For further information, you might want to contact Mediscope Medical Information, Ltd., 243 East Shore Road, Manhasset, NY 11030 (telephone: 516-627-1931).

SOME OTHER LISTS

How about your Social Security number? Do you know it from memory? I recently made it a point to learn mine, after more than 35 years of continuous use. Make note of your hospital and medical plan numbers and other health insurance information—including the companies that issued the policies and a way to contact them. Are the policies good overseas? Did you include the name and address of your family physician in case there is need to contact him or her?

We go on a trip for pleasure, to explore the world, to find joy in nature and the ingenuity of man; and we really don't want to think about health and accidents and medical emergencies. We like to ignore it particularly when we're young, because we are totally invulnerable during those marvelous years when we backpack, sleep under trees, and don't think of looking much past the first wonder of traveling. But most experts warn us that young people are especially vulnerable, because of the very ways in which they travel.

Some years ago, the Peace Corps did a study in which they found that the major causes of injury and hospitalization for younger people who travel were accidents involving automobiles, motorcycles, and bicycles. Coupled with the fact that they also tend to ignore preventive health advice and immunization, young travelers make up a large percentage of the more depressing statistics of travel—from emergency surgery to Montezuma's Revenge. Of course, many of us smug, older folks don't do much better.

A FEW MORE WORDS ABOUT VACCINATIONS

Though I touched on the area of immunization and the risks of disease at the beginning of this chapter, I'd like to go into a bit more detail at this point. For overseas travel, especially to the undeveloped and underdeveloped areas of the world, it is perhaps the most important health subject of all. As a matter of fact, those of us who ski or mountain climb or jog or play tennis at our nearby playground or resort would do well to keep our tetanus record up to date!

Not only is it a good idea to begin getting your vaccinations a long time in advance, because some of them may require more than one shot, but the most practical reason of all is the potential reaction to those shots. You don't want to be traveling while your arm is aching from the last typhoid booster, and you don't want to arrive carrying a debilitating fever from the cholera shot. Some of us, of course, have very little reaction. I was once convinced that my body was so filled with vaccines, antibodies, chick embryos, and cultures, that nothing in the world could ever affect me again, no matter how large the needle, no matter how close to departure I took the shot. It was only to prove me wrong that my body rebelled at my last smallpox vaccination, and my arm swelled up to twice its normal size one day later.

On a trip that we planned to take some years ago, the public health bulletins indicated that we would have to take a series of shots that totaled 17 injections in all. Oh, we were off to the dregs of the world, we were, and the doctors prescribed the worst: yellow fever, cholera, plague, typhoid, typhus, tetanus, and 15 as-yet-unnamed other diseases. And so, for the months prior to the trip, we scheduled our vaccinations to allow the body to recuperate from each assault of the needle. At least, all of us did but one! He decided to wait, and, unbeknownst to the rest of us, he took his 17 shots in a period of about two to three weeks. One morning he walked into the office looking yellow-green. The next four days before the trip he did not show up at all. Since almost all of my stories have happy endings, I should also say that he did show up for the departure, though his arms remained sore for a week afterwards.

THE CERTIFICATE OF VACCINATION

There is really only *one* certificate of vaccination that is accepted in all parts of the world. It is issued by the U.S. Public Health Service, and it's approved by the World Health Organization. There is no other accepted form, no matter what you are told by your friends, relatives, loved ones, or travel agent. Since the form also gives the information as to vaccine batch numbers, manufacturer, and validating stamps (where needed), you can be sure that your trip through Health and Immigration at your destination will proceed more smoothly. There have actually been cases of travelers being turned back or quarantined because of incorrect or incomplete certificates. There was a time, also, when the certificate was exactly the same size as the U.S. passport, and I stapled my immunization record onto the back cover. Unfortunately, the new passports are somewhat smaller, and I now carry both documents separately. Being a natural worrier, it gives me one more thing to worry about losing.

One of the best tips I can give you about your international vaccination certificate is to make certain that the date is written out completely—for example, 2 December 1980. If your doctor uses the normal U.S. abbreviation of 12/2/80, most countries in the world would assume that your vaccination had been given on February 12 rather than December 2, since almost

INTERNATIONAL CERTIFICATES OF VACCINATION

AS APPROVED BY
THE WORLD HEALTH ORGANIZATION
(EXCEPT FOR ADDRESS OF VACCINATOR)

CERTIFICATS INTERNATIONAUX DE VACCINATION

APPROUVÉS PAR
L'ORGANISATION MONDIALE DE LA SANTÉ
(SAUF L'ADRESSE DU VACCINATEUR)

TRAVELER'S NAME—NOM DU VOYAGEUR

ADDRESS—ADRESSE (Number—Numéro)   (Street—Rue)

(City—Ville)

(County—Département)   (State—État)

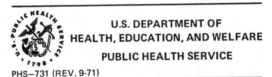

U.S. DEPARTMENT OF
HEALTH, EDUCATION, AND WELFARE
PUBLIC HEALTH SERVICE

PHS—731 (REV. 9-71)

International certificates of vaccination (approved by the World Health Organization)

everywhere else in the world, the *day* is listed first and then the month is given. It is 3:00 A.M.; you have traveled eighteen thousand miles; the airport is at 120°F. You can see your friends waiting for you on the other side of the glass barrier, and you are trying to convince an Immigration Officer who speaks very little English (and you do not speak Urdu) that the vaccination is *not* out of date. "It was December 2, Officer, *not* February 12."

WHICH SHOTS
DO YOU TAKE?

It is not my purpose here to list each and every vaccination, detail all the series that are available, outline the potential reactions, or warn the pregnant, the infirm, the infants, and the allergic. That is what doctors are for, I suppose, and there are facts and figures available to those of you who might want to pursue the subject for an upcoming trip. It would take an entire book to describe the various injections, inoculations, and vaccinations, as well as their histories, side effects, and contraindications. Two of them are in my travel library, and you may well want to add them to yours. Both are well done, and both are complete in every detail:

- *Health Information for International Travel* (HEW Publication No. CDC 79-8280), available from the U.S. Department of Health, Education and Welfare, Public Health Service, Center for Disease Control, Atlanta, GA 30333. The booklet is free, and, in addition to information about vaccination and prophylaxis, it also has tips about water, food, insects, swimming, allergies, and other health problems.

- *The Traveller's Health Guide* by Dr. Anthony C. Turner, Senior Overseas Medical Officer of British Airways (second edition, May 1979). It's available from Bradt Enterprises, 409 Beacon Street, Boston, MA 02115 ($6.95 plus shipping). It also gives some excellent travel/health advice on a number of subjects, in addition to a complete rundown on the pretravel immunizations you might need.

Just about the time that this book was going to press, another large, extensive guide was published. It's a fairly complex and complete guide to the medical services in 23 countries, and it carries listings of doctors, hospitals, ambulance services, consulates, and police emergency numbers. In addition, it gives first-aid procedures and some language translations for medical emergencies. For those of us who have to carry our medicines or drugs with us, there is a detailed section on the generic names of most medications. Though the book seems overwhelming at first, it may be of value to travelers who have serious medical problems and might need help overseas. It's called *Traveling Healthy* by Sheilah M. Hillman and Dr. Robert S. Hillman (Penguin Books, New York, 1980, $7.95 in paperback).

For those of us who like to see our information given to us more succinctly and in an easy-to-read form, IAMAT publishes a World Immunization

Chart and a Malaria Chart, as a part of its service to travelers. They are simple to follow and give a country-by-country listing, outlining the areas that require immunization against cholera, infectious hepatitis, plague, smallpox, typhus, yellow fever, and the routine immunizations such as diphtheria, polio, tetanus, and typhoid/paratyphoid.

AND A FEW
FINAL TIPS

Some vaccinations are required—smallpox is still needed for some areas though it has theoretically been wiped out. Keep in mind, also, that the validity of some vaccinations is for a very short time: cholera vaccine, for example, has a validity of from six days to six months only, while yellow fever vaccine lasts for ten years. If you travel constantly, you will learn to keep your immunization record up to date, even if you have not taken a trip in some months. Those of us who travel on a moment's notice don't like to be reminded that our typhus shot is due. For the rest of us, we come right back to allowing ourselves enough time before the trip to complete any series we might require.

Before you decide to go, check with your doctor about the need for a shot for polio or infectious hepatitis. It will probably depend upon the area into which you're traveling. The two books that I noted earlier can be of tremendous help to you. The IAMAT charts provide the easiest use of this information.

I would like to recommend again that you keep your tetanus boosters up to date. They can be just as necessary after a puncture wound or auto accident ten miles from your home as in a foreign land. I keep my typhoid boosters current as well, in spite of the fact that many of my trips are to noninfectious areas. I keep remembering the typhoid outbreaks in Switzerland and in Scotland not too many years ago, and both countries are noted for sanitation and cleanliness. Incidentally, once you take your first two-shot series, you'll need a booster shot only every three years.

ALLERGIES TO DRUGS

Be sure to ask your doctor about possible side effects, especially for immunization prescriptions that must be taken throughout your trip. The best example of this is the antimalaria pill that is prescribed for many parts of the world. For several trips, my doctor had been prescribing chloroquine—

27

once a week for two weeks before leaving, one pill each week on exactly the same day during the trip, and then a continuation for six weeks after return. (It takes that long for any larvae to hatch, and discontinuing the pills could be a disaster.) I found, though, that just like Atabrine during World War II, the chloroquine was giving me sleepless nights and a slight case of nausea in the mornings. At that time I discovered that there were, indeed, alternate pills that could be taken. I settled on camaquin, which my druggist says is exactly the same as chloroquine, but he cannot tell me why I no longer suffer from side effects when I take the pills. There is also a drug that is taken daily (Paludrine)—a pain in the neck for some of us, but a blessing for those who find it easier to remember a daily pill than a weekly one.

There are some among us who cannot or will not take any drugs, nor will they accept vaccination or immunization. The best advice I can give is that it would be wise to check the consulate or embassy of the country to which you are traveling. In some rare cases, a certificate of exemption will be issued, but keep in mind that other countries will just not allow you in without the proper forms signed and validated. The alternative, if you insist, is possible quarantine and return to the point of departure.

Of course, no matter what precautions we take, there will sometimes be occasion to see a doctor while traveling here and abroad. The hope is that we can protect ourselves well enough *before* we go, so that any visits to the medical profession in a strange world will be of no real import. There will always be the normal upsets of our digestive systems, sometimes from food that is too rich or too different, rather than badly spoiled. There will always be sunburn or a cut foot on a pebbled beach. These are things we cannot anticipate.

On a trip to Greece, I had been working out in the sun for several days, protecting myself as well as I could with hat, long-sleeved shirt, and sunglasses. Nevertheless, my body began to break out in a blotchy rash. It could not be the sun, I thought, because it spread throughout the protected areas and it itched like mad. Since I was convinced that I was dying of some dread disease, a curse of ancient Greece, I was referred to an English-speaking doctor by my client's secretary. After I had undressed, he looked at me dolefully, saying nothing. I waited for the diagnosis. Finally, he laughed, slapped me on the back, and said, "There is nothing wrong with you. Americans can't be sick. You drink too much milk!" I still don't know what caused the rash, but it left me two hours after my visit to the Greek doctor.

GETTING IT
ALL TOGETHER

On Packing ... a Personal Emergency Kit ...
and What You Should Not Take at All ...

At the end of all the airline trips, the game of "baggage roulette" begins (unless you've carried your lightweight bag right with you and placed it under your seat on the plane). Anxious arriving passengers, we among them, scan the carousel as it grinds its way around the snaking course, carrying with it the clothing, gifts, assorted small animals, skis, and other paraphernalia that rejoin us at the journey's end. And, while we stand and wait, convinced that our bag is not among them, even though we checked in early, we look carefully at the amazing array, the astounding variety of luggage that passes before us.

There are Gucci and Vuitton matched sets; standard American Tourister; Val-Packs; Samsonite; green and tan and yellow leather tote bags; canvas duffel bags; knapsacks; half-opened cardboard suitcases that have given up their strength during the trip; luggage tied with cord, with tape, with baling wire; round and square and oblong makeup cases; boxes of pineapples from Hawaii or oranges and grapefruits from Florida; and a box or two that requires that you wrench your neck to read:

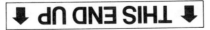

This experience alone would make me look askance at the travel books that tell you just what type of luggage to take on your trip and just what clothing you'll need. But there is a still more basic reason. None of us can lay down one rule that will fit every situation. We are all different, thank goodness, and we all wear different clothing for different occasions. Some of us feel cold when others are comfortable in light cotton shirts. A cameraman I work with appears early in the freezing 10°F morning, dressed only in a T-shirt, while I am huddled in a parka, a down vest, and winter underwear. Needless to say, he and I pack differently for our trips.

The type of journey you are taking is important to your packing needs. If you are planning a trip to Yosemite National Park, you certainly would not be packing the same way as if you were off to Paris and a round of three-star restaurants. Traveling by car requires different thinking than do trips that are to be made by plane or ship. The length of the trip is, of course, most important—a shorter one might allow you to carry everything right on board a plane with you, eliminating the need to check your luggage at the airline counter.

COVERING THE CLIMATES

We find that on many of our trips we are exposed to *both* cold and warm climates in a span of three weeks or less. Or sometimes we leave New York in the dead of winter when frost forms on my mustache, but our destination is a steaming jungle 12 hours away. This is a common experience for the many travelers who go from cold to warm climates for their vacations. Sometimes a more difficult mental predicament presents itself when we are leaving the warmth of the summer to end up in a frigid climate. It is not easy to pack in uncomfortable heat and humidity while projecting to a time, just a few hours later, when our overcoats will feel good. These are the times when most travelers are apt to pack too little clothing or to select the wrong things to take along.

It all goes back to some of the first advice that I gave: Plan ahead and find out as much as you possibly can about your destination, keeping in mind that many travel books do fabricate just a little bit. (My *Synonym Finder* offers the word "lie" for "fabricate"—just a bit too strong in this case.) Some places in the world have three seasons—wet, rainy, and monsoon. Yet the guidebooks make light of the fact that you may be slogging through three feet of water when you want to get out of your hotel and into a taxi. In other places, the

30

acknowledged rainy season is from April to October, but you get there in November and it is pouring. Your hosts merely shrug and say, "I can't understand it. This is very unusual!"

And so, since you can expect that every place you ever travel through will have "unusual" weather, unlisted holidays when stores are closed, strikes, computer reservations problems, and a variety of other dilemmas, what you pack, how you pack, and what you carry with you may well help you bridge these occurrences more easily.

WHAT TO CARRY
WITH YOU

Before we approach the "real" packing and the suitcases for heavy clothing, I'd like to make some suggestions about the things that you should be carrying right on your person, and add to that a few tips about an over-the-shoulder travel bag that can go right along with you on the plane. The same suggestions hold true for train or car travel, by the way. Even steamship travel has changed somewhat since my grandmother packed a huge steamer trunk out of which she lived while aboard the ship. It had one section in which she could hang her clothes, and drawers on the other side for smaller items. It has been in our basement, unused, for 20 years now, and we still talk about opening it some day to find out what is packed away inside.

• Always keep your passport right with you. This goes for visas and any other important travel documents you may need.

• Your international certificate of vaccination should also be on your person.

• Don't forget driver's license, traveler's checks, credit cards. Some countries require an international driver's license.

• Carry a small amount of your money in dollars, in denominations of one, five, and ten. These can be put right in your wallet. (I will cover this more fully in Chapter 23, on currency and tipping.)

• Take earplugs and eyeshades for sleeping on aircraft.

• Take a ball-point pen. If you're traveling overseas, you'll constantly be asked to fill out entry forms, Customs declarations, hotel registers, and passport information. Pens that fill with liquid inks tend to leak aboard aircraft.

• Unless you're traveling domestically, there's no need to take airmail stamps with you. They won't be of any use in another country.

A PERSONAL
EMERGENCY KIT

On each and every trip, I take with me an over-the-shoulder bag with several compartments, one of them filled with my traveling "office," another section with maps and travel literature; the center section acts as an "emergency kit" that is stocked for almost any situation. In fact, on a long trip a few months ago, the catering service went on strike just as the aircraft was about to be supplied. As a result, no food was put aboard. (Of course, this is sometimes a boon on today's carriers!) Out of my emergency kit came granola bars, raisins, peanuts, and three mountain climber's emergency food packs. My seat-mate and I were saved!

In addition, I pack an ordinary airline flight bag with other supplies that I think I'll need on the trip, and I stuff it down at the bottom of my suitcase. What goes into it depends entirely upon personal travel preferences, the type of trip, and the eventual destination. If I'm traveling in the United States, I certainly need not pack extra toothpaste or soap. Overseas, the requirements change dramatically. On certain trips, the center section of my black carryon bag might hold extra clothes, and, on other trips, it might include an emergency supply of quick-energy foods. But whatever else the bag contains, the one thing that I must tell you about is my horseshoe. I never travel without my horseshoe. It's the first thing I pack, and I'm not even superstitious!

In 1963 I opened an office in Rome, and my landlord gave me the horseshoe as a good luck token. He had been given the horseshoe by *his* first landlord, and now he was passing it on to me. Well, though I don't believe in omens, witchcraft, or magic, I just don't like to take chances, and so I have carried it with me on every trip since then. Once, while going through Manchester, England, on my way to Spain, the Customs Officer, digging deeply in my bag, came up with my horseshoe, and, without blinking an eye, he said, "My, you must have a lovely horse out there somewhere!"

THE AUTHOR'S PERSONAL KIT

Before writing this chapter, I took that black bag of mine and emptied all the contents on the floor of my office. After all, I had never really done an inventory of all the items I had collected over the years and which I firmly believed were necessary, each and every one of them. The pile began to grow; my coworkers peeked through my office door, convinced that I had gone insane; and I made my list, not knowing whether to laugh or be embarrassed. For whatever it's worth, here it is:

- Food, including peanuts, mountain survival packets, granola bars.

- Business cards for my offices in New York and London.

- Three small sewing kits taken from hotel rooms.

- One sewing kit with braided thread of about one hundred colors. (I have only found this in England, and it's a marvelously ingenious invention.)

- Scissors.

- Scotch tape.

- Memo pads.

- Stationery and envelopes.

- Combination bottle opener and corkscrew.

- Small toothbrush (two, in fact), with paste.

- Earplugs.

- Eyeshades.

- Soft slippers.

- Safety glasses.

- Ice scraper for car windshields.

- Band-aids.

- Tissues.

- Comb.

- Paper clips.

- Three plastic bags.

- Pencils, pens.

- Address book with people and places (collected over 35 years).

- Large piece of heavy twine. And, herein, lies a story.

The day I made my inventory, I repacked everything and left on a trip. As I took my suitcase out of the taxi and gave it to a skycap, the handle broke (for the twenty-seventh time!). Undaunted, I took my trusty twine and tied the handle to the case, while the skycap stood by and looked amused. I looked up at him, smiled, and said, "That was the way my grandmother came over from Europe—with all her suitcases tied with rope." He thought for a moment, nodded his head, and laughed, "You sure can learn a lot from those old ladies!" The handle has since been fixed, and the new length of twine is again in the black bag.

But I am not finished. I have only emptied two of the sections in the black bag. Bear with me—the strangest contents are yet to come:

- Do Not Disturb signs in English, French, and Japanese, since they never seem to be in my hotel room when I want them. As a matter of fact, I'm not even sure the Japanese one says Do Not Disturb, since I can't read the language anyway.

- Booklet of maps of the United States.

- Extra passport photos.

34

- Fingerprint sheet from the New York City Police Department, since some countries require it for entry.

- Good Conduct letter from the same agency attesting to the fact that I am, in no way, a "perpetrator," nor have I ever been, to their knowledge.

- Cardboard parking disc from the city of Brussels, something they use there instead of meters. (You never know when you'll be without one just when you need it!)

SOME OTHER USEFUL ITEMS

Of course, you may not need all of this. It is my own personal security blanket, just as yours will be. So, on a more practical vein, here are some of the things that *you* might consider packing before you go:

- Medical supplies that you may need on your trip. Prescription drugs should be right on your person. And don't forget aspirin, band-aids, suntan lotion, cosmetics.

- Toilet paper. In many parts of the world, it's good to have your own supply. Much of the globe is without paper entirely, while the other half seems to use waxed paper backed with sandpaper.

- Extra prescription glasses.

- Sanitary napkins or tampons. These are not available in some countries.

- Small travel alarm clock (as quiet as possible). I just do not trust hotel wakeup calls, especially when I'm off on a 6:00 A.M. flight the next morning.

- All-purpose antibiotic. Have your doctor prescribe one before you leave. We use ampicillin.

- Vitamins. We always have some with us for the areas where we can't really eat much of the food that's around.

- Remedies for motion sickness, diarrhea, the common cold.

35

• Insect repellent. The airlines do not permit passengers to carry aerosol sprays aboard aircraft, however.

• Shower cap.

• Spot remover.

• Sewing kit with multicolored thread.

• Tube or plastic bottle of detergent for washing your clothes when no laundry service is available. It's a good idea to check your itinerary for the number of "laundry days" you have. Most hotels with "one-day" service do not do laundry or dry cleaning on weekends.

• Folding plastic hangers with little clips at the end that can be hung right over the shower bar. As a substitute, take some inflatable hangers with you. I also include a length of nylon line, in case there is no shower bar.

• Electric transformer and the specific types of plugs you'll need at your destinations. There are some small, compact kits now available in department stores and specialty hardware shops. Be sure you check with your travel agent or tourist office before leaving. Many electrical appliances, such as hair dryers and electric razors, cannot be operated without adapters or transformers. Either the voltage ranges from 160 to 230, or the cycles are 50 rather than 60—or the plug is a three-prong type that you've never seen before.

• Small, throwaway flashlight. Though I am all for recycling and reuse, and firmly against anything that must be thrown away after use, this is one exception that works well. It is small, compact, and easy to carry right along with you. Since I live in hotels or motels a good part of my life, I am firmly convinced that one night I will lose my sense of direction and end up in a closet while on my way to the bathroom. For diabetics and older people who can bruise themselves dangerously in a darkened room, the flashlight is a must.

Of course, there will be more—your own personal toothbrush, razor, manicure material, deodorant, and whatever else it is that fills your medicine cabinet at home. Make sure you repack liquids in plastic bottles and then put each one into a small plastic bag that is tied at the top. Don't forget a folding umbrella, and you might even carry a lightweight folding rain poncho in your over-the-shoulder bag. I even carry a roll of heavy-duty fabric tape, in case my bag is torn in transit.

PROTECTING YOUR FILM FROM X-RAY

Of course, you will be taking a camera and plenty of film. Extra film is not available everywhere, and, in any case, you'll be paying a premium price for it in most places. Carry with you only what you need immediately, then pack the rest of the film in your locked suitcase. However, keep the film and loaded camera handy enough so that you can remove it from your hand luggage when you go through airport security.

When the low-intensity X-ray machines were first installed, signs were posted stating that they would not hurt your film or tape. Those of us in the professional film field never believed the signs, and it turned out that we were right. The X-ray is additive, and if the setting is too high when your film passes through many of the detectors on a trip, the film will fog. Not only are some machines indeed set too high in intensity, but information has now been reaching us that some airports are also X-raying *checked* luggage! In that case, the new lead-lined packets or lead-lined paper will help protect the film you've packed in your suitcase.

At one time, we used to meet tremendous resistance when we asked that our film and cameras be all hand-inspected rather than sent through the machine. We had to call supervisors, threaten lawsuits, cajole, smile a lot, and shake our heads negatively while being told that it was "all right." Finally, they learned that we did have a point. Film was fogged, tapes garbled, the memories of trips taken by friends ruined by the X-rays which just weren't working properly that day.

A personal friend of mine had 27 rolls of film fogged irreparably as she came out of Mainland China and into Kai Tak Airport in Hong Kong. You will now find that, in most places of the world, security agents will smile and examine the film and camera by hand. Take my word for it. It's worth the extra trouble.

THE HEAVY PACKING

A long time ago, I decided that I would just not keep going through my wardrobe to make a new selection each time I was off on another trip. I bought

37

two dozen blue cotton shirts (with epaulets), a gross of black cotton socks, and a gross of black woolen socks; and I had the same shoes made for me in Hong Kong—twelve pairs of brown and twelve of black. It is much easier these days, for I have no choices to make; and, with the addition of some of the "better" clothes that I might need on the trip, such as jackets, ties, and trousers, I can pack and be out of the house in 20 minutes. Of course, one dark morning, knowing where everything should be, I packed quietly and tiptoed out of the house, only to find as I arrived on location a thousand miles away that I had taken one brown shoe and one black shoe! It occurred to me that I had a pair just like that at home!

The American Society of Travel Agents (ASTA) suggests that packing has three main objectives, and I agree wholeheartedly:

- To protect clothes in transit.

- To make them easily available when you arrive.

- To make them easy to repack.

WHAT KIND OF SUITCASE?

About the best advice that anyone can give you is to choose a suitcase that is fairly lightweight, with soft sides, made from a durable material, and easy to close. When it's packed, you should ideally be able to handle it yourself for short distances, since many places in the world just do not provide assistance at airports or hotels. Yet, in other places the arrival of a tourist brings "instant people" to assist with your bags, children, and dogs.

I personally use a soft-sided folding suitcase that can be hung on a rack when I arrive or laid out on the bed for unpacking. It holds a huge volume of clothing and other articles, and it has withstood 50 or more trips, with the handle only breaking twice. Now, having discovered this superb article for travel, I find that it is no longer being manufactured! You may have your own personal favorite; possibly it even has wheels on it so you can take it where you need to go without help.

Whichever suitcase you use, make certain you check with your travel agent or airline about baggage allowances. Domestic carriers and American overseas airlines have now replaced the weight limitations with a regulation

.

that limits only the size and number of pieces that you can take with you. The airlines of other countries, however, still limit baggage according to weight — 44 pounds in economy class, 66 in first class. Should you have more pieces than you are allowed, or should the weight exceed the limit, you will be charged excess baggage costs.

I assume that you will choose your wardrobe carefully, since you probably don't own the one-shirt, one-shoe, one-sock array that I do. Keep in mind that, in some of the places, you may need more formal clothes, a bathing suit, *comfortable* walking shoes, an extra sweater (even if the climate is supposed to be mild), and perhaps a pair of gloves for a cool evening. Then, after you've gotten all your clothes together, try to hang them out where you can see them. Display the underwear and shirts and socks on the bed, put all your suits or dresses nearby, and see if things coordinate. Possibly you've taken too much. Go over the number of days in your head and, just as you did earlier, walk through the trip. What will you be wearing in the morning, for sight-seeing, at lunch, at the ballet or opera, for dinner with clients or friends? Remember that if your trip will cover several cities, you can wear the same thing in each city — which brings me to our "polyester" society.

There is no doubt in my mind that synthetic fabrics are easier to take care of, easier to launder yourself, easier to pack, with fewer wrinkles when you unpack. Unfortunately, I am convinced that synthetics are just the wrong fabrics to take on most trips. They get cold in cold weather, don't breathe in hot weather or in the tropics, and, even if they do launder easily, they're just not as healthy nor as good as natural fabrics — cotton and wool. Later on I will talk about the layer theory of dressing or undressing — for example, wearing a pair of cotton socks over which you put a pair of wool socks for colder climates. If the weather turns warm or you arrive in the tropics, the wool socks come off, leaving only the cotton on your feet. In any case, it is a personal choice, and I find that I have been much more comfortable since I began letting my body breathe again.

MORE PACKING TIPS

There are a few tips that I'd like to pass on to you, since it is impossible to give you specific information on just what order to use in putting your clothes into your particular suitcase. Just pick and choose the ones that seem helpful.

• If you use a folding soft-sided bag, as I do, the clothes are put in right on the hangers, allowing you to take them out quickly at your destination and hang them in the closet.

39

- Put all your items in separate plastic bags by category: underwear, socks or panty hose, shirts or blouses. They can be removed easily and then repacked quickly. Too, you need never take them out of the bags if the hotel dresser drawers are slightly seedy or even moldy.

- Include some extra plastic bags to be used as laundry bags or for items that you might pick up along the way.

- Also include a soft, foldable canvas bag that can be used to carry home the gifts and souvenirs that you're bound to buy.

- Put your shoes in plastic bags. (Though some suggest using fabric "mittens" for the shoes, I have never had any problem with plastic.)

- Inside each shoe, use the available space to pack small items such as gloves or socks, panty hose or extra film.

- Pack the heavier items first, using the sides and bottom of the bag to pack your plastic bags of accessories, your shoes, belts, emergency kit, travel books, extra film, or an extra purse.

- If you are using a suitcase that does not really let your clothes lie flat while packed, and you decide to roll them, make sure they're rolled tightly. Close the buttons, zip the zippers, and smooth out the wrinkles as you roll.

When you're finished packing, paste a business card or some other identification with your name and address on it on the inside cover of the suitcase. You might also include your intinerary, so that the airlines can find you if your luggage is lost. Lock the suitcase—a psychological thing at best, for anyone can get into any suitcase if he really wants to—and make sure you have an extra set of luggage keys with you, kept separate from the first set.

Regulations now insist that you also put a label with your name and address on the *outside* of the suitcase. However, there is a tip to keep in mind when you do so. When the rule went into effect, the professional burglars and thieves among us came up with a marvelously clever idea. If they drifted around the airports and managed to make note of the names and addresses of the people who were traveling, then the homes from which they had just come would be empty and tempting. It is wiser to put your name and address on an identification tag that can fold over and thus hide the information. Or you can do what we do—put the name and address of your *business* on the label. It serves the same purpose, and it's a lot safer. Incidentally, I will discuss lost luggage in Chapters 14 and 21.

WHAT YOU MAY NOT PACK

There are, unfortunately, some items that are illegal and extremely dangerous to take with you if you are traveling by air (courtesy Civil Aeronautics Board, Washington, D.C.):

• Aerosols: polishes, waxes, degreasers, cleaners, insect spray, deodorant spray, hair spray.

• Corrosives: acids, wet cell batteries, cleaners.

• Flammables and explosives: paints, thinners, lighter fluid, liquid reservoir lighters, fireworks, flares, loaded firearms. Small arms ammunition for personal use may be *checked*, but not carried aboard.

• Radioactive materials.

• Compressed gases: protective-type sprays, oxygen cylinders, divers' tanks (unless empty).

• Book matches or safety matches may only be carried on your person.

WE'RE OFF!

You have changed your mind at least 15 times about the extra shoes; the suitcase will not close easily, in any case. What results from the packing session will be your own very personal luggage, filled with only the things that reflect you. One friend of mine always encloses his favorite dry cereal, since he is convinced that his trip will be ruined without it. A client of mine travels with a large, round, awkward, ugly green hair dryer, and she cannot be talked out of it. After all of our 28 pieces of film equipment have come out and are loaded in the van, her hair dryer finally makes its lonely appearance on the belt. I have

41

learned to live with it. For all I know, you cannot (will not) travel without your teddy bear. The trip is yours, take what you will. See you at the airline baggage carousel. Mine is the one labelled:

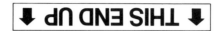

5

SITTING, RUNNING, JUMPING, STANDING, JOGGING, SLEEPING, AND BREATHING

... A Brief Guide to Staying Fit on the Trip

This is a difficult chapter for me to write, for I am basically against any exercise that does not come as a normal part of my job, my hobbies, or the hyper personality that keeps me moving all the time. I would much prefer to turn over again and get some additional sleep while I hear the pounding of the heavy-footed runners outside my window each morning. For me, the word "tennis" merely means "tennis elbow," and I have been convinced for years that too much exercise merely destroys the muscle tone that I spent years building up as a boy.

Nevertheless, I grudgingly admit that my job keeps me physically active, and what I do not receive from deliberately punishing my body, I do get by accidentally punishing it through long trips, mountain climbing with film crews, and running to another location. And since this is the time for confession, I must also admit that when I keep active, I do feel better and more alive. This is even more true when I take one of my long trips on a plane or in a car, and my muscles have a tendency to fall asleep, while my brain becomes numb and my blood congeals from lack of movement.

We are, for the most part, a "sitting" society, in any case. We sit in our chairs at the office, be it an executive chair or a secretarial one; we sit in cars to travel two miles to the supermarket; we sit in the theater, on the beach; we spend endless hours on the couch or in a club chair watching television. We sit while we read about how sitting is making our heart muscles weaker, that our blood is standing still in little pools while varicose veins are painting patterns down our legs, and that our muscles are gradually atrophying. And so we go on vacation—and we sit some more.

We sit in deck chairs on ships while our ankles swell from lack of circulation, a condition that was at one time called "deck ankles," and we sit in cars, and we sit in airplanes. The technology has not helped at all, for the flights seem to get longer and longer, though the jet is touted as speeding us there more quickly. Nonstop planes soar from New York to Tokyo, or from Honolulu to Fiji. And, where the airline seats were once billed as comfortable and roomy, additional rows have been added to almost every jet, giving the traveler little room to move either left or right, front or back, up or down.

Our knees touch the seat in front of us, our elbows lock with those of our neighbors, and the child behind us makes matters worse by flapping the tray table up and down, up and down. We don't even have room enough to turn around and complain! It's no wonder that we arrive at our destination feeling as though we had traveled the eight or ten hours packed into the overhead baggage rack.

Of course, a long trip is a long trip, and you expect to arrive tired and with your body rhythms a bit out of sorts. But there are things that any traveler can do to make the trip more comfortable. You can make yourself more relaxed and at ease, not only through exercising and keeping yourself from melting into an immobile mass, but by learning how to plan your trip properly, how to relax before and after, how to sleep, drink, and eat properly, and how to select the right clothing for the journey.

BACK TO THE BLUEPRINTS

I spoke of planning earlier in the book, and I will probably speak of it again. So much of your pleasure (or pain) on a trip will depend upon how well you have planned it all. And, barring the usual vicissitudes brought about by the fickle finger of Fate, it will pay off . . . at least, most of the time.

If at all possible, plan to take your trip during what you might consider the "normal hours." I realize, of course, that what is normal for me is not normal for others. I am a "morning" person, and my wife is a "night" person—an incompatible marriage for over 33 years! She would like to do everything at night—read, travel, see films, have dinner. I, in turn, am up at the crack of dawn and totally exhausted by three in the afternoon. Everyone in my office is aware of my three o'clock slump. I am, in fact, famous for it. Since I am the author of the book, however, we will consider "normal hours" as the daylight hours. For me and for people like me, the curse of today's travel is the night flight or the 24-hour continuous journey on a jet that is traveling faster than our grandmothers could ever have imagined.

DAYTIME FLIGHTS VERSUS NIGHTTIME FLIGHTS

I suggest that you check with your travel agent and with the airlines before you rush off to your vacation retreat on the first available transportation. It is not always possible to travel by day, certainly. But investigation will frequently uncover a way for you to get there more easily and feeling a lot better on arrival than you did on the last trip. In Chapter 11, I will discuss the problems of the executive who must travel at night, but for now, I assume that we are on vacation. What's the hurry?

A FIRST WORD ABOUT JET LAG

• Try to travel on daytime flights if you can, especially on relatively long trips. Most flights to Europe leave at night and arrive the next morning, with the traveler squeezed into a new time zone and the body rebelling every step of the way. (See Chapter 7, on jet lag.) It is possible to travel the Atlantic via a day flight to England, arrive about 9:00 or 10:00 P.M. Greenwich time, have a light dinner, sleep, and then make the first flight in the morning to Athens or Rome or Brussels. I have done this time and again, and it makes all the difference in the world.

• On the really long trips—to Australia or Fiji or Manila—try making a one-day stopover in a place like Hawaii. If it's vacation time instead of business, try making the stopover for two days—it gives you time to unwind and spend a few days at a comfortable hotel and then continue on to your destination a bit more relaxed. Of course, you will still be tired when you get to Australia, but you will not begin your vacation totally exhausted.

PLANNING STOPOVERS

When we make our long air trips now, we generally try to make *two* stops on the way—for example, San Francisco and Honolulu. It's a far cry from our first trip from New York to Sydney back in 1961. It was to be Alitalia Airline's inaugural flight from Rome to Sydney (Alitalia was a client of mine), and we were invited along.

On Monday night, we started out from New York to Rome, where the festivities were to begin. The plane had engine trouble over the Atlantic, and we turned back to John F. Kennedy Airport. We were put up at a hotel in Queens, and that night the city suffered a severe blackout, so the air conditioning did not work on the hottest day that summer. Our luggage was still aboard the plane, so we had no change of clothes. We left again for Rome on Tuesday night, arriving at Fiumicino Airport about 11:00 A.M. on Wednesday.

Because we obviously are masochists, we still did not rest, but ran into town to have luncheon with Roman friends at a lovely restaurant in the Piazza Navona. The inaugural flight left for Sydney at 4:00 P.M. Wednesday, fully packed with invited guests, including us—sated with wine, Roman sunshine, pasta, and good Italian cheer.

Every four flying hours, the DC-8 made a stop, and more inaugural festivities were held. The hours passed; the nights were four hours long, the days of equal length. We danced in Teheran at midnight (their time), had breakfast in Bombay after a quick stop in Karachi, lunch in Phnom Penh, a midnight shower in Darwin Airport (the first in four days), and arrived in Sydney *at 7:00 A.M. on Friday* (their time). Did we feel tired? Of course not! Our spirits were high as the jet circled the field three times, the normal maneuver for an inaugural flight. We drove into town—and immediately went sight-seeing! Needless to say, the collapse came soon afterward.

The change is quite evident. The last time we visited Australia, our fourth trip, we stopped over in San Francisco and then again in Hawaii. We arrived in Melbourne at 11:00 A.M., just in time to "take a nap." We discussed dinner plans, some favorite restaurants we might visit that evening, some friends we might call when we awoke a few hours later. Then, tired but happy to be back in that most marvelous country, we fell asleep.

When we awoke, I looked at the clock. It read somewhere around eight o'clock—just enough time to shower, dress, and have dinner. There was one problem. It was eight all right, but it was eight o'clock the next morning. We had slept through the night, for nearly *20 hours*. And so, famished, but feeling well rested, we ate what is called a "drover's breakfast" of steak, potatoes, eggs, bread, and coffee. Though I may be ahead of my story, for I plan to cover arrivals later in the book, one important tip stands out when you travel by air on a long flight: *Rest for 24 hours after your arrival.*

CLOTHING

Your comfort on a trip, whether on a plane, train, or in a car, also begins with what you wear. I find that my most difficult trips are the ones on which I must be dressed as a businessman, because of a meeting on the other end or because I am being met by my clients or more conservative friends. There is nothing more uncomfortable for travel than a shirt and tie and the restrictions of a jacket or vest. My wife tells me that she avoids any binding clothes at all—tight underwear, snug boots, or even belt buckles that can press too tightly into the body. As a result, if we have the time on the other end—time to check into the hotel with an hour or two to spare, time to unpack our clothes—we dress comfortably for the trip and then change at the final destination.

This philosophy, however, can have other side effects. I have found that when traveling as a "businessman" I can get more satisfaction from the airlines or hotels should a problem arise—double-booking, computer breakdown (one of the great excuses of our civilization), no record of a room reservation, lost luggage, and so forth.

Dressed in comfortable blue jeans and a blue denim work shirt with a leather jacket, I am likely to be taken for an aging hippie or an itinerant hobo, and therefore may not be listened to. I remember, some years ago, checking into a Chicago hotel after a three-day car trip from New York, accompanied by my wife, my luggage, and my German shepherd, who had had a rather bad time on the trip. He had been stung by a bee at one rest stop and got an emergency antihistamine shot from a kindly Ohio veterinarian. His nose was puffed up and covered with calamine lotion to ease the pain. As if that were not enough, the next rest stop was littered with America's rubbish, and the poor dog stepped on a broken beer bottle, this time treated by an Indiana vet. His right front paw was bandaged from sole to shoulder, and he sat forlornly in the lobby as we checked in. Everyone made a long detour around him, for obviously he was rabid with fever.

The desk clerk was cool, officious, snide, and wishing that we would just get out of his clean lobby. It was the dead of summer, it was steaming hot with the humidity that flows off Lake Michigan, and we were shown to our room. It was in the old section of the hotel and was not air-conditioned, though a window opened up over the main street of town. Overall, our treatment was obviously reflecting our appearance.

I knew the room had to be changed if we were to enjoy our stay in Chicago. Nothing else was available in town, since there were four conventions all being held at the same time. Fully aware of the desk clerk's attitude toward us when we had checked in, dirty and unkempt from the three days on the road, I showered, put on my best suit, knotted a tie, wore brilliantly shined shoes, and went down to the reception desk again. It was as though I were another person, possibly even the president of the United States. The room was changed without trouble. After all, a "businessman" might well be a steady customer!

Some of this attitude has disappeared in the United States and Canada with the easing of social rules, for almost everyone wears blue jeans today — some with more chic labels than others, but blue jeans nonetheless. But much of the feeling still exists in South America and Europe, where formality continues to be the norm. However, I prefer to travel in comfort and worry about the problems as they arise.

Here are some things you might consider when you plan your wardrobe for the trip:

- Wear comfortable, loose-fitting clothing and, by all means, wear comfortable shoes. Your feet and ankles may swell when you fly for more than a few hours, and if you've taken off your shoes, you may have trouble getting them back on at the end of the flight.

- Take along a pair of soft slippers to wear when you take off your shoes. At one time the airlines gave them to passengers, and I still have several sets, but I have not seen them aboard for some years now. This is also good advice for trains and buses.

- Carry an extra sweater, soft jacket, or turtleneck pullover, in case the plane or train gets chilly. I mentioned earlier that, when we're packing and the outside temperature is 95°F, we have a tendency to ignore *where* we are going and how we are going to get there. Remember your destination—and remember that the plane is pressurized at an altitude of five thousand feet. Also keep in mind that various sections of the plane can be hotter or cooler than other sections. Trains can be drafty, and part of your trip may well be through mountainous terrain with severe temperature drops outside.

EXERCISE AND MOVEMENT

My friend, cameraman Joe Longo, took an extended trip from Los Angeles to Tokyo aboard a jumbo jet. The usual amenities (such as they are) were completed, the meal service was over, the movie long finished, and still there remained interminable hours to be passed. His seat-mate, a Japanese traveler who spoke no English, stood up, bowed, and made his way past Joe into the aisle. There, calmly, quietly, with great dignity, he began to remove his clothing, placing each item neatly on an empty seat. When he had stripped down to his undershorts, he put on a colorful kimono, sat down on the floor directly in the aisle, and began to do his exercises!

At this point, the traveler had an audience of hundreds, and the attention of a flight attendant who pleaded with him (in English) that he was blocking the aisle and that it was firmly against IATA regulations. Not understanding a word, the gentleman continued to do his exercise, changed back into his clothes, and politely made his way back to his seat.

Now, I am not recommending that you go out and buy a kimono for your next flight, but the Japanese gentleman had the right idea. By getting up and moving around, he was treating his body with care and with consideration. Not for him the stagnation of the blood and the gradual dissolution of the muscle tissue!

EXERCISE WHILE FLYING

Even if you are against formal exercise, as I mostly am, it is wise to get up several times during your trip just to move around. Your circulation will

49

improve, your head will remain clear and alert, and your arrival will be less of a trauma, even though you have traveled through eight or ten time zones.

A few years ago, an airline finally admitted that flying long trips can be tedious and tiring, and that it is not all caviar and champagne and dancing in the aisles. Scandinavian Airlines (SAS) developed a clever and valuable little pamphlet titled *Exercise in the Chair;* it is reproduced here with their permission. The pamphlet was so popular, in fact, that a complete book was published soon afterward, to expand upon the need for exercise and movement not only in travel but throughout the entire "sitting" society in which we live. It's called *SAS In-the-Chair Exercise Book,* by Dr. Folke Mossfeldt and Mary Susan Miller (Bantam Books, New York, 1979, $3.95).

Essentially, SAS has merely carried through to its logical conclusion the idea that it's very beneficial for you to keep moving during flight. Even if you are not inclined to "jog on the spot," or do shoulder, head, and hand turning, or foot rolling, their point is well taken: Don't sit still during the entire trip! Even if you get up to visit the lavatory several times or to see what magazines are left in the rack, the movement is beneficial. The last "sport," incidentally, is an interesting game. Invariably, the popular magazines like *New Yorker, Time, Newsweek,* and *Vogue* are gone, leaving you reading material such as *Miniature Golf Magazine, National Cat Fancier,* and *Arizona Highways.*

Just try walking—walk to the back of the plane, look at the faces as you pass them. Walk back to your seat and look at the backs of heads. But get up and walk! Once in your seat, do the suggested SAS exercises or make up your own. Twist your ankles and wrists, move your shoulders up and down, wiggle your toes.

Knowing that I like to move around on a long trip, I try to choose a seat on the aisle rather than near the window. I know that most people like to "look out" and see the scenery, but, at thirty-seven thousand feet over the ocean, the scenery, such as it is, can be awfully boring. Having an aisle seat permits me to move around without having to climb over my neighbor's lap, across his food tray, and over his excess baggage in order to get to the lavatory or to the magazine rack. On the other hand, it does subject *me* to my neighbor (or his child) climbing over me, my food tray, and my own excess baggage each time he wants to visit the rear of the plane or his relatives seated all the way on the opposite end of the row. This generally happens, of course, just as I have completed my exercises and fallen asleep with exhaustion.

I should mention one final thing for exercisers—and especially those of you who pound past my window at dawn each morning. Not only do the airlines not allow dancing in the aisles, but they also frown upon jogging.

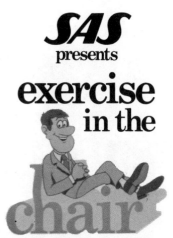

SAS
presents
exercise
in the
chair

An inflight exercise program for the air traveler. No. 2

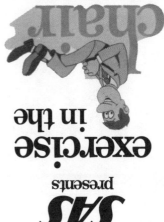

An inflight exercise program for the air traveler. No. 1

exercise in the chair

presents

SAS

SAS *SCANDINAVIAN AIRLINES*

SAS takes care of you...

The human body is made for movement and therefore functions better with regular exercise.

Nowadays, we often spend long periods sitting down–in an office chair, at the theater or in a comfortable airline seat–when our freedom of movement is somewhat restricted.

SAS takes care of you in every possible way, and have produced a special series of exercise films with useful advice on how to keep fit and active even while seated.

We offer you this simple but effective exercise program to help keep you fresh and alert during the journey and bring you to your destination in top trim both mentally and physically.

...and helps you take care of yourself

Here are some additional tips on how to keep fit after you have returned home:
- exercise your whole body two or three times a week by running, walking, cycling, swimming, or similar activity
- keep your limbs and joints in trim with regular exercise sessions – rhythmic movements using the full range of the joint
- at work and play exercise your muscles as often as possible, trying to use a rhythmic pattern of movements in which the muscles are tensed and relaxed alternately for equal periods

Exercise is good for you

We all know that exercise does us good. But did you know that the right sort makes all this happen:
- the heart pumps better because the heart muscle receives a greater supply of blood
- the lungs breathe more effectively because the breathing muscles work better
- the quantity of blood increases, supplying more oxygen to the various parts of the body
- the blood vessels are stimulated
- the joints retain their mobility and vitality
- more muscle cells are produced, which in turn receive more nourishment

In terms of health this means that you are in better condition, have greater vitality and resistance to the type of illness and disease commonly associated with a sedentary life.

Folke Mossfeldt Medical Adviser

In-flight exercise program offered by SAS

51

Exercise program No. 1

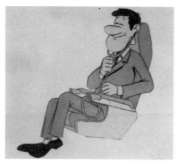

1. Jogging on the spot.
A warming-up exercise.
It makes sense to warm up properly before strenuous exercise. Use simple, rhythmic movements, engaging as many muscle groups as possible. "Jog on the spot" by raising your heels alternately as high as possible. At the same time raise your arms in a bent position, and rock rhythmically forward and back as when walking. Continue 1–3 mins.

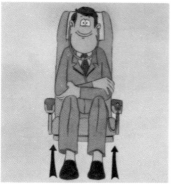

2. Raising on the toes.
Improves blood circulation to the legs.
Sit with elbows on knees, bending forward with your whole weight pressed down on the knees. Lift up on toes with the heels as high as possible. Drop heels and lift toes. Repeat whole exercise 30 times.

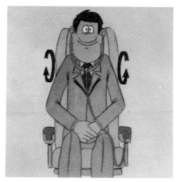

3. Shoulder rolling.
Stimulates the joints, relaxes shoulder muscles.
Joints thrive on regular motion. Smooth, rhythmic movements "lubricate" the inner joint. Move the shoulders gently and rhythmically, at intervals, describing large circles in both forward and backward directions.

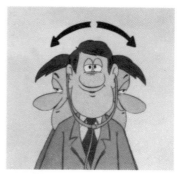

4. Head turning and nodding.
Stimulates joint capsules and cartilage in upper spinal column.
It is important to regularly activate the joints to the full extent of movement. Occasionally do the following: Turn the head the fullest extent to the right. Nod a few times. Do the same toward the left. Repeat the entire exercise six times.

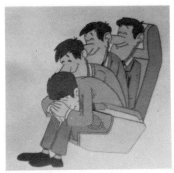

5. Forward bends with stomach in.
Stimulates bowels and blood circulation.
Stimulate blood circulation and improve the digestion with this exercise: Draw the stomach fully in. Drop the trunk forward while lifting the front of the feet high up. Place the toes back on the floor, relax the stomach muscles, and raise the body upright again. Repeat some thirty times.

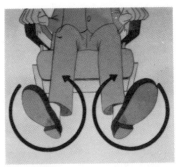

7. Foot rolling.
Stimulates the ankles.
Exercising the ankle joints now and again by rolling the feet in large circles to the full extent of their movement is a valuable form of stimulation. Repeat 15 times in each direction.

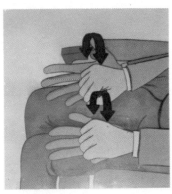

6. Hand turning.
Stimulates the wrists.
The cartilages and joint capsules in the wrists also need stimulation. A good way to achieve this is to turn the hands all the way over and spread the fingers. Return hands to original position and relax them. Repeat 15 times.

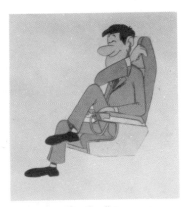

8. Knees up against the elbows.
Speeds up blood circulation.
Now and then, preferably at regular intervals, one should increase the blood circulation by setting to work large groups of muscles. This is one way: Drive the left and right knees alternately up toward the opposite elbow. 15 times in each direction.

STOSP 983 013   LITHO IN DENMARK · INTERPRINT A/S

Exercise program No. 2

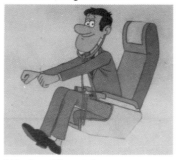

1. Rowing while seated.
A warming-up exercise.
This warm-up session takes the form of an imaginary "rowing" action. Stretch the arms forward while bending the upper body forward for a rowing "stroke". Lift the forward part of the feet right up, then press down the toes, draw in the arms and at the same time move the body backwards, completing the "stroke". Repeat the exercise for 1–3 mins.

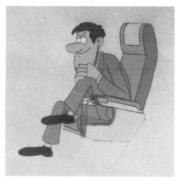

2. Alternate knee raising.
Speeds blood circulation.
In this exercise we speed up the blood circulation and flow by lifting the left, right and finally both legs in succession. Grasp the hands together and "pull". Repeat the exercise 10 times each for left, right and both legs.

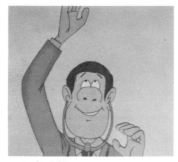

3. "Apple-picking".
Stimulates the shoulders.
The shoulder muscles and joints are stimulated by alternately and rhythmically stretching up the arms as if picking fruit from a tree. This exercise is alternated with a rhythmic movement of the shoulders forward and back, holding them in a dropped, relaxed position. Repeat exercise 10 times with each arm and the shoulders.

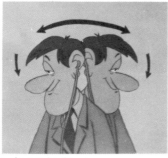

4. Alternate head turning.
Stimulates joint capsules and cartilage in upper spinal column.
Bend the head forward (chin against the throat). Keep the chin against the throat and "bend" the head backwards. Turn the head as far as you can to the right and nod 3 times. Return the head to the front. Do the same toward the left. Repeat the whole exercise 10 times.

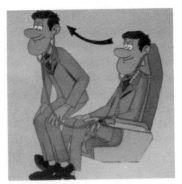

5. Rising and sitting.
Improves flow of blood to legs and blood circulation.
Speed up circulation and stimulate the passage of blood to the legs with this exercise: Gently rise upward or attempt to rise, with or without the help of the hands. Sit down again and lift the toes. Repeat exercise 30 times.

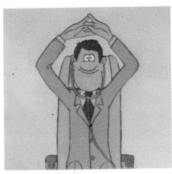

6. Double arm-swings.
Stimulates the shoulders.
To stimulate the muscles and joints of the shoulders and elbows: Sit with the hands clasped. Swing the arms gently, rhythmically upwards and backwards, stretching them while turning the palms upwards. Bring the arms down again and relax. Repeat the exercise 10–20 times.

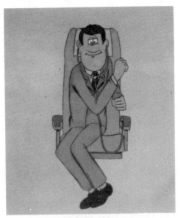

7. Slalom while seated.
Stimulates the blood circulation.
"Slalom-skiing" improves the passage of blood to the legs and stimulates blood circulation. Sit with the heels as far out to the right as possible, with both the hands on the same side. Lift the heels right up and swing them all the way over to the left while swinging the arms over in the same direction. Repeat the exercise 30 times.

8. Relaxation. Muscle control.
We often tense various muscles unnecessarily for short or long periods, sometimes without realising it. Training muscle control and relaxation technique helps counteract this and is beneficial in other ways. Try this exercise: Sit fully relaxed. Breathe evenly and gently using so-called "diaphram" breathing. This involves "filling" the stomach when breathing in, which is an active motion. On breathing out, which is a passive motion, the air is slowly released and the body sinks into complete relaxation.
In order to become aware of the difference between tensed and relaxed muscles, helping to avoid unnecessary tensing, as mentioned above, practise alternately tensing and relaxing various muscle groups. Repeat the exercise until you feel heavy, pleasantly relaxed.
Folke Mossfeldt Medical Adviser

AND FOR CARS, BUSES, AND TRAINS

The rules are, of course, exactly the same no matter which form of travel you might choose. The cross-country trip by automobile can be just as exhausting as a long plane trip. The difference is that you can stop at your leisure. (It is rather awkward to go outside the aircraft for a short walk, though I must admit that I have been tempted to ask some especially noisy children to "go outside and play.")

Of course, people who travel by car and who have children or German shepherds or any other variety of pet are fairly lucky. The tedium of man's ingeniously designed, monotonously boring highways is not for them. The children demand their stops for bodily functions that make themselves felt from their mouths down to various other parts of the anatomy, and the dog must be walked at intervals of every hundred miles or so. This allows for involuntary movement and exercise. And, just when everyone is settled again, the car suddenly needs to be gassed and oiled—all too often, considering today's prices for fuel.

For car travel, as for trains, buses, and planes, it's a good idea to exercise and stretch your legs every once in a while. It's amazing how quickly the head can clear. Stop every hour or so to stretch your legs, move around, look at the scenery, get some fresh air. And, of course, all this makes sense unless you are with a driver (or are the driver yourself) who refuses to stop, so that you can "make time."

A friend of mine used to drive to Florida from New York twice a year. Once, we made the mistake of going along with him. For three days he refused to stop unless it was absolutely necessary. If he could have had a lavatory in the car, he would have had it installed, along with a tank truck that would gas us up as we moved. He just didn't want to stop. About the second day, I asked him the reason, for, after all, we were all going on a leisurely vacation. Growling as he accelerated, he answered, "If I stop, all those guys I passed on the road back there will now pass me!" We flew back to New York.

EXERCISE ABOARD SHIP

As I mentioned earlier, even the cruise ships have their "sitters," and ankles are just as likely to swell at sea as they are in the stratosphere. But aboard today's liners, the opportunities for exercise are sophisticated and complete. In doing the research for this book, we came across ships that included swimming pools (indoor and outdoor), massage facilities, saunas, jogging decks, supervised exercise classes, a gymnasium fully equipped for almost every form of structured exercise, vibration machines—and superb kitchens that feed you too well and send you back to work it off again.

With the popularity of jogging on the increase, some ships have set aside separate areas for the runner who must get that mile or two into the day's activities. (Other ships discourage joggers since the sound of pounding shoes carries into the cabins below.) But keep in mind that these decks sometimes have stairs as a part of the "track," they are much more crowded than the country lane you've been running on every day, and they generally have one additional hazard besides the pitch and roll of the ship. I speak of the wind.

It has been described by shipboard joggers and runners as having the same effect as running uphill. On one side of the ship, the wind may be at your back, making you feel as if you are well on your way to an Olympic gold medal and a new world's record. As you round the stern or bow (depending, of course, upon which way you are running), the gale hits you in the face, and suddenly the pleasure is gone. Of course, some runners merely stay to the leeward side of the ship, running back and forth over the same route. Some of us would applaud this good sense, while others would call it cheating, I know.

One woman I know ran every day of her cruise, rain or shine, wind or calm. She did it for 60 straight days, as the ship made its way from continent to continent, from the West around the globe to the East. When the ship finally docked, she had not missed a single day. She now boasts that she has run completely around the world!

FOR THE SLEEPERS AMONG US

All of us, even the exercisers, must rest, and the long plane trip is a good excuse to shut the world out, to read, to think, and to sleep. It is a time, too, to moderate your intake of food and alcohol, to cut smoking to a minimum, and to try to drink plenty of fluids while aboard. I will cover all of these in later chapters, especially the subject of how to avoid some of the airline catering, but for now, just a mild word of warning is sufficient. I have been aboard charter flights where the alcohol flowed continuously from takeoff to landing, and I have no pleasant memories.

I can sleep easily on planes, and I know that some of you cannot. There is little that can be done about it except to try to make yourself as comfortable as possible. If you are lucky enough to have two empty seats beside you (a feat that is becoming rarer and rarer in airline travel), take out the arms of the adjoining seats and make yourself a bed. Some arms lift up, some do not come out at all. Those of us who travel a great deal have become expert at removing any and all airline seat arms.

Place a blanket on the seats, put two or three pillows near the window, take off your shoes, lie down, strap one seat belt loosely around your waist, and cover yourself with another blanket. Put on eyeshades, plug your ears with some kind of material, either plugs or cotton, and sweet and pleasant dreams to you. Of course, if your legs are sticking out — for the seats are still not large enough for you — people will keep hitting your toes as they pass in the aisle. If your head is on the aisle, it works in reverse. Either way, I am not promising a night's sleep on a Beautyrest mattress. We do the best we can.

Even if all the seats are taken, you can sleep more comfortably in your own seat by using the eyeshades and earplugs, taking off your shoes, and stretching out as far as you can with your feet under the seat in front of you. You may think that this last bit of advice is impossible, since you have stuffed your overnight bag, two sacks of oranges, and presents for the grandchildren under that seat. But keep in mind that stowing all of your carryon luggage in that area is required by law only during takeoff and landing. Therefore, when it's time to sleep, just move them out and under your legs, then stretch into the space you've just cleared.

Once you are asleep, I guarantee you that your neighbor will then want to climb over you to get to the lavatory. Following that, the flight attendant will lift your eyeshades to ask if you would like to eat what is passing for food that particular day; or, failing that, headsets will be passed out for a movie you didn't want to see in the first place; or, just having fallen asleep again, the plane makes its final descent for landing. You may not be well rested, but at least you're there!

6

"STOP THE SHIP—
I WANT TO GET OFF!!"

*Hopefully, an Unnecessary Treatise on
Motion Sickness and How to Deal with It*

Almost every traveler who returns from Italy comes back with stories about the *Italian* drivers! Even by the tone of their voices, you can tell that the word *Italian* is in italics, and the description is completed by an exclamation point. Having had an office in Italy for three years, and having worked there for many more, I can safely report that the Italian driver has been unfairly maligned to the point of slander. The Italian driver, in spite of what your friends report, is one of the best drivers in the world.

There are, of course, qualifications that must accompany this statement. Every Italian child wants to grow up to be a racing driver. Thus, the automobiles made in Italy have their speedometer needles set to read ten kilometers when the car is standing still. This allows every driver to feel that the car is going that much faster through the entire trip, whether it be in the winding streets of Rome or out on the highway where there is essentially no speed limit. All of this, combined with the Italian *punto d'onore* or "point of honor," a special form of "macho," provides the passenger with a breathtaking experience unlikely to be forgotten. When the Italian driver signals that the car is about to turn, the car is indeed about to turn, and this is what seems to

59

confuse the American motorist, who is more familiar with the rules of the "civilized" road. This brings me to my story about my friend Marco Cicero.

We were to drive from Sorrento to Positano, down the Amalfi Drive. For those of you who have not been there, let me hasten to say that it is one of the most gorgeous roads in the world, at least insofar as the scenery is concerned. The sea stays close to your right, down a steep cliff most of the way, though some barricades have recently been installed. On the left is the mountain range that guides you all along the way but provides very little shoulder for emergencies or breakdowns. Most spectacular of all are the curves—hundreds of them—that switch back on top of one another all along the route. No straightaway seems longer than 50 yards, and the curves come one after the other, to the accompaniment of screeching tires, trucks and cars coming in the opposite direction, and the shifting of passengers' stomachs.

Marco, a superb driver, but much like all my Italian friends, had dreams of driving at Le Mans, of winning at Daytona, of being crowned driving champion of Italy, Europe, the world! But most of all, Marco was out to prove to me that the entire trip from Sorrento to Positano could be made without the use of his brakes! All turns would be negotiated by shifting gears down and then up again, and it was a point of honor to prove it to me—the American used to driving on all those straight superhighways.

Interestingly enough, he did prove it, for I am here in one piece and able to write about it. But as I was sitting in the back seat of the small Fiat, my fear soon gave way to a peculiar sensation in the pit of my stomach. Each time we turned, my insides turned, and each time he shifted down to a lower speed, another hairpin curve swung us 180 degrees down and around the roller coaster highway. To put it mildly, I had motion sickness—the single worst case that I have ever had and that I ever hope to have. Today, I still smile wanly when I think of it. And I must admit that I went back to the Amalfi Drive several weeks later and tried the same thing—only this time I was the driver (point of honor, macho, call it what you will). Marco was right. I could drive the entire Amalfi coast without once using my brakes! But as the driver, in another seat and not subject to the long swaying of the rear of the car, not only was I *not* sick—I was *exhilarated!*

WHAT IS
MOTION SICKNESS?

Nobody really knows what motion sickness is (which is a great way to begin a chapter about it). Oh, there are theories, all right, but there are theories on perpetual motion, cholesterol, and the exact date of the end of the world. The interesting thing about motion sickness, however, is that you don't even have to be in motion in order to feel the symptoms! Some years back, there was a first, highly acclaimed performance of Cinerama in which the theater audience was taken on a trip aboard a roller coaster. It was so realistic that many in the audience felt nausea and vertigo, and I found that I had closed my eyes during one horrendous drop.

Motion sickness does not even confine itself to the major forms of travel—ship, plane, car, or bus. There is a story that Lawrence of Arabia got "seasick" aboard his camel! The best theories seem to blame a combination of sensations from the inner ear and the eyes as the chief cause. If conditions are right, regardless of where you are or what mode of transportation you're using, the familiar symptoms of paleness, a cold sweat, headache, or dizziness— and, in its worst stages, nausea and vomiting—will make themselves quite evident to the victim.

The inner ear is the organ of balance. I remember that several years ago I had been flying rather constantly for almost three weeks. The continuous change of altitude, the pressurization of the cabins in the jets, the tension of the business travel all combined to infect my inner ear. I discovered it one morning when I awoke in my hotel room, sat up in bed, and then fell down in a heap, unable to keep my balance even while sitting up. To say the least, I was frightened, but it passed in a few moments, and the doctor told me what was wrong. Since then, I have heard the same stories from flight attendants who go through the same routine I did, but on a regular basis.

Researchers have found that quick, jerky movements of the head will affect the balance mechanism of the brain—thus my reaction to the driving of my friend Marco. But the inner ear is not alone in this scenario; there are times when the eye may have much to do with how you feel while traveling. If your visual reference lurches while you're traveling—rough seas, for example—you can become ill. Later on, I'll try to give you some tips about what to do and what not to do. Some of them may help you. Notice that I said "may" help you—for everything that I've stated so far is not an exact science. Other factors play a role, and here is where researchers cannot agree as to cause and effect of motion sickness.

Some of us (myself included) are terribly susceptible to odors, especially foul ones. This has not helped my work in some of the world's worst slums (where I breathe through my mouth), and it has caused what might easily be called motion sickness on several occasions. The air in a jet becomes stagnant and foul-smelling, even with separate smoking and nonsmoking sections. This is particularly true on the longer overseas flights. There's just no way to "open the window" and let in some air. Some of the more civilized airlines will have the flight attendant go through the cabin and spray air freshener from time to time. Of course, for someone with a large, sensitive nose such as mine, this is merely exchanging one foul odor for another one, albeit sweeter.

EATING AND OVEREATING

What you've eaten will also affect how you feel aboard the plane or ship or car or bus or train. Before you go, eat lightly. Stay away from fried or greasy foods. Do the same when once aboard if you have a tendency to suffer from motion sickness. Strangely enough, the body maintains itself, and you will survive without overeating before and during the trip. Looking at some of America's junk food served on the road these days, a traveler can get motion sickness by just sitting still at the table!

But overeating and the various forms of gluttony can begin right before your trip, as well as once you're aboard. The bon voyage party is probably one of the prime causes of illness during travel, especially if it's held just the night before you walk up the gangway or make your way groggily to the airport. Too much alcohol, too many cigarettes, too much food, an early-morning bedtime before an early-morning flight, and you wonder why you don't feel too well at the very beginning of your trip to paradise!

Heat can also affect the traveler adversely, and later on in this chapter you'll notice that I recommend plenty of fresh, cool air when I discuss the specifics of traveling by ship or car. Here, too, I am a sufferer. Heat affects me, while cold does not. I do everything I possibly can to keep my body temperature at a comfortable level.

IS IT ALL IN THE MIND?

And finally, there is a culprit that really makes a fool out of experts and scientific researchers—our own mental state before and during our trips. Each of us reacts differently, each of us approaches a journey with a different attitude. Anxiety, fear, trepidation, foreboding can all make us ripe for the onslaught of motion sickness.

My mother was a terrible traveler. She managed to get sick in airplanes, in cars, in trains; and the only ship she was ever on was the one that brought her to this country as an infant. Even though I figured that she was only two years old when she arrived here, she still regaled us with horror stories of the seasickness aboard the ship. I was always convinced that her problem was mostly psychological, and, on one trip, she proved it to me.

She was on her way from New York to Tulsa to visit my younger brother. Sitting in the airport lounge, she was a bundle of nerves. Her hands moved rapidly and jerkily, her eyes darted around the room, her lips looked dry, and there was nothing we could do to comfort her. The captain of the plane walked by and noticed her. He must have been a kind man, certainly he was an observant one. "Well now," he smiled, "where are you headed today?" My mother, trembling, managed to stutter the word "Tulsa." She also gave him a weak smile. "Look," he said, leaning over to speak to her, "when you get aboard, come visit me in the cockpit. I'll show you how we fly the plane." And, with that, he went aboard. My mother's eyes followed him as if she'd fallen in love again.

Several hours later, my mother telephoned from Tulsa to say that she had arrived safely. "How was the trip?" I asked. For five minutes she went on about the pilot and the crew, how they had looked after her, invited her to the cockpit when she didn't show up voluntarily, pampered her, talked to her, and generally made it the most memorable flight she'd ever taken.

"Didn't you get sick?" I asked. It was as though I had given her a new thought, something that had never entered her mind before. "Sick?" she repeated, "Sick? Why should I have gotten sick? It was such a nice flight."

And so there are, indeed, many factors that create this strange and unusual affliction, not the least of which is the human mind. Some of us get sick sometimes, some of us are never affected, while others of us find that we react differently on every trip. There are sufferers of motion sickness who eventually get their "sea legs" and some who never do. It is with little consolation that we learn that Britain's renowned Lord Nelson got seasick each time he boarded his ship and set out to sea.

ABOARD THE SHIP

The rules before sailing are the same as for any trip—keep your system as clear as possible for several days before you go. Rest as much as you can, eat lightly, and cut down on your intake of alcohol and tobacco. Most large vessels today have a stabilizing system that keeps them fairly smooth during most of the trip, and you might keep that in mind when you or your travel agent are booking the trip. The larger the vessel, the calmer the ride. I recently completed a series of films for Holland-America cruises, and I was astounded at the stability of today's ships.

• Remember that some seasons will bring you rougher seas than others.

• Choose a cabin, if you can, that is near the waterline and as close to the middle of the ship as possible if you are normally a victim of motion sickness. You may not have a porthole, but today's liners are air-conditioned, and cabins are quite comfortable (though small) almost anywhere on the ship.

• If you're on the outside of the ship, make sure the cabin has plenty of ventilation, and, again, try for a cabin down near the waterline rather than up near the top deck. The roll of the ship will be less severe.

If you should feel that you are becoming seasick:

• Get plenty of fresh air.

• Lie down in a deck chair with your eyes closed.

• Don't overindulge in the marvelous buffets that the ships now offer. Eat lightly, get your "sea legs," and then keep your diet light throughout the cruise.

• If you really feel that the end of the world is fast approaching, visit the ship's doctor. All modern liners are well equipped for emergencies. There is even an injection that can be given to help you overcome motion effects. The name of the drug is Pmenegran (manufactured by May & Baker, Ltd.), promethazine hydrochloride, and it's given intramuscularly. The patient is also advised to lie down and rest for two hours after the injection. It's FDA-approved, by the way, and it can be found both here and abroad.

• If you're on a small yacht, a fishing vessel, or a pleasure craft, you are more apt to feel the pitch and roll of the boat. Keep busy if you can—do anything to get your mind off the feeling. If you can't keep active, keep your eyes on the distant horizon. Remember, the rapid or jerky movement of your head or eyes is what is causing the uneasiness. The horizon moves more slowly than anything else around you.

ABOARD THE PLANE

Now that the jet has almost completely replaced the piston engine plane, airsickness has become less common. Gone are the good old days of wondering not only how fast you were traveling from east to west, but also how fast you were moving *up and down!* Announcements about turbulence are less frequent, and, when they do occur, the altitudes at which we fly seem to even them out somewhat. Certainly, there are rough flights, and the edges of widespread thunderstorms can buffet any aircraft in the vicinity. But if you fly a great deal, I think you will admit that these occurrences are rare.

Still, some people do suffer aboard planes, for whatever reasons—many of which we have already covered. To help make you more comfortable when on a flight, here are some tips that you might follow:

• Wear loose, comfortable clothing. This is a tip that I gave earlier, but it can help to keep you at ease during your flight. No tight belts, girdles, shoes, if possible.

• Keep your alcohol intake down, both before the trip and aboard the plane. Since alcohol is a depressant, you would expect that a drink or two in the cocktail lounge before a flight would just put you to sleep. Right? Wrong. At least, sometimes it's wrong. Though some travelers find that a few drinks make the trip an unmemorable blur, for others the alcohol actually creates a *feeling* of motion in some nerve centers, thus hastening the onset of motion sickness.

• The ventilation systems of today's aircraft make the air exceedingly dry. Make certain you maintain your fluid levels when you fly. We find that we always arrive at our destinations feeling thirsty and dried out. Stewardesses use special creams to keep their skin moist because of this problem.

• If you have a tendency to feel queasy on a plane, choose a seat in the middle of the aircraft and in line with the wings. This is especially appropriate for the jumbo jet, where the midsection is large, roomy, and fairly stable.

• Keep your smoking to a minimum. The oxygen up there is thin and dry enough without adding to your problems.

• If you feel the symptoms of motion sickness, relax with your seat pushed back as far as possible, close your eyes, loosen your clothing even more. It may help if you also direct the overhead blower toward your face, to give you the feeling of cool air passing over you.

• Eat little or nothing. As I said before, you will survive the flight without partaking of airline food. In some parts of the world, in fact, not eating might improve your chances of survival!

• One added tip: Many drugs to relieve motion sickness have side effects (discussed later in this chapter). If you are a flier who is going to rent a car after the trip, be particularly careful about the drugs that you take. Some may make you sleepy enough to affect your driving adversely.

IN THE CAR OR BUS

The story of my Italian friend gave you some indication as to a few of the problems you might encounter when traveling by car. You may also remember that I did *not* get carsick on that second trip down the Amalfi Drive. A driver never (or hardly ever) gets carsick—because of his or her position in the car and because the driver's eyes are constantly on the distant horizon of the road. Too, the driver is the one person who must sit up straight, with head held firmly atop the neck, thus avoiding the jerky movement that the passengers must sometimes endure.

• If you have a tendency to get carsick, don't sit in the back of the car. Sit up front with the driver.

• In a bus, don't sit over the wheels, which are the bumpiest part of the vehicle.

• Keep the air conditioner on or open the windows.

- If you're in a station wagon, particularly one of those long models, don't sit backwards in the rear seat in the well.

- Focus your eyes on the distant horizon.

- Don't read while you're in the car. Even looking down at a road map can bring about motion sickness. It's interesting that this phenomenon happens only in a car, not in a plane.

And, of course, there's one bit of advice I can give that relates only to a car and just couldn't be done on a ship or on a plane. If you're getting dizzy or nauseous, stop the car! Or convince the driver to stop. I realize that I could not have convinced my friend who drove with us to Florida, but possibly your friends are more humane.

AND FOR ALL TRAVELERS

There are a great number of drugs that have been developed for travelers who fear they'll get motion sickness or who actually develop the symptoms on every trip. Some of them work, and some work only for certain people. Some of them have severe side effects. Some are sold over-the-counter and carry proprietary names, while others are sold only by prescription. The best advice I can give you before listing several of these drugs is to warn you to check with your doctor before you take off on your trip. The important thing about *all* of them, however, is that they must be taken *before* you begin the journey. Once you've been stricken by motion sickness, they just won't work.

The most common are the antihistamines, such as Dramamine, Bonine, and Marezine. They have a mild, sedative action, but that also means that they can cause drowsiness. Keep it in mind if you have to drive or be otherwise alert after you've arrived at your destination. Their only advantage is that they can be purchased over-the-counter without a doctor's prescription. (Though some of us would say that this is a disadvantage.)

There are two stronger and more effective drugs that have been tested these past years, including some testing on astronauts. Indeed, many of the intrepid travelers into space from the United States and Russia suffered severe cases of motion sickness both in space and after returning to earth. In fact, several have become sick while waiting in the capsule as it floated in the sea before pickup by the aircraft carrier. One astronaut, it is told, survived space and the capsule intact, only to become violently ill aboard the ship that was carrying him home! You can begin to see what illustrious company we're all in when we feel ill while traveling.

In any case, the astronauts were given a combination of a drug called scopolamine and one of the amphetamines (such as Dexedrine). Both drugs must have a doctor's prescription and both can have severe side effects. These can include everything from diarrhea to faintness and headaches, as well as creating psychological dependence. It is important—in fact, it is critical—that you see your doctor for advice. There are believers among us who think that much of the drug dependence can be eliminated by properly planning the trip, proper diet beforehand, and by avoiding alcohol and tobacco.

There are, indeed, experiments going on across the country to find a way to avoid the use of drugs in travel. Some researchers on the West Coast have been trying biofeedback and have been testing the *psychological* responses to motion sickness rather than concentrating on the physical symptoms. It is a wise and practical path that they are following. For I am totally convinced that my own ease of traveling comes from the constant repetition in my life of getting aboard a plane so often during the year. I was, at one time, a "white-knuckle" flyer—I was frightened of planes, and I dreaded the takeoffs and the landings. Psychologists tell us that if we keep repeating the experience of flying, we will eventually become used to it, more familiar with the strange surroundings of space and the feeling of drifting seminoiselessly from departure point to destination. For some of us it has worked, and I assure you that it will work for some of you. But for the others, I am terribly sympathetic; I, too, have felt the queasiness and the discomfort while on my way from here to there. Of course, today I laugh at those times. But they were not funny when they happened.

I am reminded of a story that was told by my wife's father, Max Adams; it was humorous around the dinner table and among friends and is quite amusing to me even now. I am glad I was not on his ship, however. It all took place before the Great Crash of 1929, when cruise lines (steamships) advertised the most elegant way to travel from New York to Florida. Not by train, of course, and airplanes didn't get you there in two-and-a-half hours. How? By sea. By ship, by liner, by luxurious, ocean-going vessels that would wine you and dine you all the way down the Atlantic coast, and take you to the warm climate of Miami Beach in a way that you would always remember.

Max, his family, and four friends decided that it would be the vacation of a lifetime if they cruised to Florida over the New Year's holiday. What a marvelous way to anticipate New Year's Eve: champagne, ship's whistles, dancing—something out of Hollywood and the flapper era. There was one thing that they had not counted on, however. This was December. The wind was howling, the seas were rough, the pitching of the ship sent everyone down below deck to lie in his berth for two solid days. Only one person did not get sick—Max Adams.

And so, on New Year's Eve, he donned his tuxedo, put on his paper hat, and made his way through the heaving passageways to the main ballroom. He was not alone; one waiter stood solitary guard over a totally empty room! The band was sick, the staff was sick, and all the passengers were, obviously, sick. Only Max Adams and the lonely waiter were not. It was a quiet evening, but it was a New Year's Eve unlike any other he had ever spent.

Happy New Year!

7

"DID SOMEBODY TURN BACK MY BODY CLOCK?"

On Jet Lag . . . Why and When It Hits,
and How to Minimize It

No matter years of travel

To there and then return.

No matter wise decisions

Or all the tricks I learn.

I am but merely mortal—

My clock cannot be set.

I have the time-zone syndrome;

I've lagged aboard the jet.

M. L.

The warnings come to me in two places—my head and my stomach. I have arrived. I followed all the rules along the way. I even declined the airline lunch and dug into my black bag for the picnic I brought aboard (see Chapter 13). I am healthy; I am invulnerable; I am a world traveler. I am excited; I am looking forward to meeting old friends, having dinner at a favorite restaurant in a little plaza under the olive trees, walking through narrow streets and old haunts. I am feeling fine, and I even slept for three hours on the plane. I am ready for anything—except for the jet lag!

In a short time, possibly within the first hour of arriving on the other side of the world, I begin to feel the bubbles fizzing across my forehead. Someone seems to have opened a bottle of club soda and squirted it into my brain. My eyes feel strangely dry and tight, as though a rubber band had been stretched around my head and is too tightly pressed against the retinas. Suddenly the idea of dinner in the small plaza doesn't seem quite as attractive to me; in fact, I am not hungry for the first time on the trip. The little narrow streets can wait. My friends will understand, as they have so often in the past. I had better make my way to my room at the hotel, for the bed will look terribly inviting, and so it should. I really should have thought *first* about sleeping it off. Everything else will still be there when I awaken—my friends, the dinner, the plaza, and the city itself—and I will enjoy them all even more.

If my doctor were along, he would look at me with a twinkle in his eye (I am very lucky—I still have a physician who has a twinkle in his eye) and he would say, "My boy, you simply have a case of totally incurable circadian desynchronization, more commonly known as diurnal rhythm disruption." Of course, I have been struck down again—I have jet lag.

The pioneers who crossed the Donner Pass certainly didn't have jet lag to contend with (though cannibalism can be considered more injurious to your health); and my mother and grandmother may have gotten seasick on their way over from Europe to the Promised Land, but they never experienced the symptoms of jet lag. It is a phenomenon that has come to us as a price we must pay for being in a hurry.

On the other hand, think of the pleasures and the new worlds that have opened for the tourist who generally has only a two- or three-week vacation in which to discover the rest of the universe that lies outside our door. Thanks to the speed of the jet plane, the world now has a limitless horizon. My own feeling is that jet lag is a small price to pay for the wonders I've seen in the places to which I've been fortunate enough to travel.

THE BODY CLOCK

The problem is simple, though the solution is not. Each person's body has its own rhythm—its own clock that is set to correspond with where one lives in the world, and thus with the normal rhythms of the day. We adapt to the day-night routine of our environment just as the animals do. It is one of the reasons that workers who constantly change shift—such as firemen or police or factory workers—are heard to complain that they feel "out of sorts" when their "normal" day shift is moved to the midnight tour. Their body clock just isn't ready for it. And it's not just a matter of eating and sleeping.

Our body clock controls hundreds of functions, from body temperature to heart rate, hormonal balance, kidney function, and even breathing. So long as we stay at home, the clock continues to function fairly well and with few interruptions. But when we move too quickly to another part of the world, as we do so often in this jet age, our bodies fall out of synchronization with their familiar time frame. The people who live *there* are on another clock, with their bodies naturally integrated into this schedule. We can simply reset our watches to the local time, but we can't reset our bodies. They are still somewhere back home, as our symptoms tell us only too well.

Take a look at the accompanying time zone chart. If a given city is merely one or two hours behind or ahead of your normal clock, there should be very little problem. Millions of us travel from Chicago to Denver (one time zone) with practically no effect. The same holds true for almost every short trip across the United States or Canada. But the people who live in Djakarta, Indonesia, are living their lives *12 hours* ahead of us, so you can begin to see how the problem becomes more complex when we go there. If it is noon in New York, it is midnight in Djakarta. To this basic fact add the flying time and the tension of travel and it becomes clear why you become a prime candidate for jet lag when you fly to Djakarta.

TRAVELING EAST— TRAVELING WEST

However, to see how it all adds up, let's take a simpler example. More of us travel to Europe than to Djakarta, yet jet lag affects us in much the same way and often with equal intensity. In fact, the older you are, the more severe the effects are liable to be. London is but five hours from New York (six when we are on daylight saving time). Your flight leaves John F. Kennedy Airport at 9:00 P.M. It is just past your dinnertime (and you have eaten lightly in

City	EST	PST	City	EST	PST
Amsterdam	6	9	Juneau	−3	0
Anchorage	−5	−2	Karachi	10	13
Athens	7	10	Keflavik	5	8
Auckland	17	20	Ketchikan	−3	0
Azores	3	6	Kinshasa	6	9
Baghdad	8	11	La Paz	1	4
Bangkok	12	15	Lima	0	3
Barcelona	6	9	Lisbon	6	9
Basra	8	11	London	5	8
Beirut	7	10	Madrid	6	9
Berlin	6	9	Manila	13	16
Bermuda	1	4	Melbourne	15	18
Bogota	0	3	Montevideo	2	5
Bombay	10.5	13.5	Moscow	8	11
Brussels	6	9	Nome	−6	−3
Bucharest	7	10	Okinawa	14	17
Buenos Aires	2	5	Oslo	6	9
Cairo	7	10	Paris	6	9
Calcutta	10.5	13.5	Rangoon	10.5	13.5
Capetown	7	10	Recife	2	5
Caracas	1	4	Reykjavik	5	8
Copenhagen	6	9	Rio de Janeiro	2	5
Dakar	5	8	Rome	6	9
Damascus	7	10	Saigon	12	15
Delhi	10.5	13.5	Samoa	−6	−3
Djakarta	12.5	15.5	San Juan	1	4
Dublin	5	8	Santiago	1	4
Fairbanks	−5	−2	Seoul	14	17
Frankfurt	6	9	Shanghai	13	16
Frobisher	1	4	Shannon	5	8
Gander	1.5	4.5	Singapore	12.5	15.5
Geneva	6	9	Stockholm	6	9
Glasgow	5	8	Sydney	15	18
Guam	15	18	Tahiti	−5	−2
Helsinki	7	10	Teheran	8.5	11.5
Hong Kong	13	16	Tokyo	14	17
Honolulu	−5	−2	Valparaiso	1	4
Istanbul	7	10	Vienna	6	9
Jerusalem	7	10	Warsaw	6	9
Johannes-			Whitehorse	−4	−1
burg	7	10	Zurich	6	9

To calculate the time in the above-listed cities, add the number shown (or subtract if it is preceded by a minus sign) to eastern or Pacific standard times. For example:

New York (EST) 9:00 A.M. — add 6 — Amsterdam 3:00 P.M.
Seattle (PST) 6:00 P.M. — subtract 2 — Anchorage 4:00 P.M.

(Adjust for U.S. daylight saving time (DST) — check with travel agent for other countries that observe DST.)

anticipation of your trip, have you not?). You have left in plenty of time to catch your plane, you have worried about the last-minute packing, perhaps you have not slept too well because of the excitement and, possibly, you have even traveled in from Cleveland that very day in order to make your overseas connection. You are tired, but that's OK—you'll sleep on the plane.

It is 9:00 P.M. eastern standard time at Kennedy Airport—but it is 2:00 A.M. in London and almost everyone there has been asleep for hours. Your "rest" on the plane will last five hours, more or less, and you will cross five time zones during the flight. You are going west to east, so the night will be very short. It will be daylight on your arrival in London at about 7:00 A.M. Greenwich mean time.

On the plane you will be fed a meal when the flight reaches altitude, they will screen a movie for you, interrupted every 20 minutes by your neighbor crawling across you to get to the lavatory, and you will finally get to "sleep" about three hours into the five-hour flight. (Most people can't sleep on planes anyway.) Within an hour you will be awakened, your tongue coated with lambs wool, your eyes smarting and red, your clothes feeling as if you'd slept in them, which you have—and then they'll feed you breakfast!

Now, remember, it is about 1:30 A.M. eastern standard time, and you never eat breakfast before eight. Besides which, you certainly don't feel like having breakfast after you've just eaten dinner a few hours ago. Well, it may be 1:30 A.M. for you, but it is 6:30 A.M. for our British friends and they are up and about and ready to head down to London through the fog to go to work.

Bear with me—the mounting road to jet lag is not over. You land at 7:00 A.M. London time, which is 2:00 A.M. for you, and you proceed through the civilized Customs inspection of Great Britain to find your bag among the three hundred others. Possibly, you go on your way to town and are into your hotel between 8:00 and 9:00 A.M. local time (3:00 to 4:00 A.M. your time). It is obvious, is it not, that after crossing five time zones, after a tiring five-hour flight, after the excitement and the tension and the anticipation, *this* is not the time to begin your sight-seeing or walking tour around London? Again, bear with me. There are ways to mitigate, if not eliminate, the ravages of jet lag, but we'll get to that later.

THE INTERNATIONAL DATE LINE

You can easily see the problems on a short trip to London or Paris, so just imagine the additional complexities of traveling 10 or 12 or 20 hours on a jet plane and then, on trips across the Pacific Ocean, crossing the international date line. It's like flying across the end of the world. Depending upon whether you are going east to west or west to east across that line, you gain or lose one entire 24-hour day!

When you travel west to east, you actually "gain" a day. For example, when you leave Sydney, Australia, for San Francisco at 1:00 P.M. local time, you cross the international date line and the clock (time, not body) immediately falls back 24 hours. Thus, if you go by the calendar and "real" clock, you will arrive in San Francisco *before* you left Sydney. On the other hand, if you were traveling from east to west when you crossed the date line at 12:01 A.M. on Wednesday, it would instantly be 12:01 A.M. on Thursday and you will have lost all of Wednesday forever. Crossing the date line can be a trauma for people who have to take pills each day at the same time—like contraceptive or fertility pills; suddenly they discover that they have lost Wednesday somewhere along the route!

One of our more amusing traveling companions also wondered, if you kept crossing the date line going west to east forever, would you get younger and younger? We did not answer—we were having enough trouble with normal jet lag, which brings me to the symptoms that accompany this affliction.

ADJUSTING TO JET LAG

The immediate response of the body varies from traveler to traveler. Some of the symptoms of jet lag have already been discussed and if none of them fit your particular case, never fear—I'm certain that you will have your own very individual reactions to the trip. For some, there is a bubbly fizziness in the head, a feeling of sluggishness or sleepiness. For others, there is a loss of appetite, lethargy, and a very noticeable diminishing of mental alertness and reaction time. This can be dangerous for drivers on unfamiliar roads or in countries where the drivers keep to the left. (This phenomenon, incidentally, takes place in more countries than you would care to count. Wherever the British have gotten there first, one drives on the left.) Another immediate reaction to jet lag, interestingly enough, seems to be an effect on short-term memory, and even the simplest mathematical problem seems impossible to complete. For those of us who pride ourselves on our mathematical ability, it is a severe shock to discover that computing a simple currency exchange in order to give a tip to a skycap has become a problem.

The symptoms I've described above can last anywhere from one to four days, with the eating and sleeping functions returning most quickly. Some researchers claim that it takes one day of readjustment for each time zone crossed. If this is true, you can well imagine that your trip would be nearly over before you felt that your own body clock had synchronized with that of the natives. Actually, with the simple functions returned, you will be fairly comfortable in a very few days. But other parts of the body will not have caught up. Over a hundred bodily functions are thrown out of kilter by jet lag; certain of these do not stabilize for over two weeks in some cases. It is not simply a matter of eating and sleeping—your body temperature, heart rate, blood pressure, breathing, hormonal balance, urine, blood, kidneys, and liver are all affected. Constipation is a fairly common result of jet lag (though this is sometimes involuntarily "cured" by a severe case of the Tourist Trots).

Generally speaking, the traveler going west to east seems to get the worst symptoms of jet lag. The days and nights are short and the time gets later as you progress on your plane trip. On east-to-west trips, the days and nights are stretched and the body gets a little more time to adjust to it. It means staying up a bit later until bedtime after you arrive, and it just seems to help on shorter trips. However, there seems to be very little effect of jet lag on north-to-south trips (or vice versa).

When we travel to South America, we find that the airline schedules demand that we leave at some ungodly hour like midnight and travel all night to Quito or Bogota. The flight is generally about eight hours long and we arrive tired (and happy) during the morning rush hour. Strangely enough, though we have traveled on a long journey and have fallen victim to normal fatigue, we do not ever suffer the unpleasant consequences of jet lag. A short nap, and we are ready for lunch—for lunchtime in Quito is lunchtime in New York, and our body clock has told us that we are ready to eat.

WHAT CAN YOU DO TO ELIMINATE JET LAG?

The answer to eliminating jet lag is exactly the same as the answer given to the problems of motion sickness. Nothing really. Your body clock will revolt no matter what you try to do, but there *are* ways to ease the ravages.

For one, try to travel during hours that are normal for you, if at all possible. For example, let's go back to the New York–London trip that I described earlier. Instead of a flight that leaves at 9:00 P.M., we simply move the flight time 12 hours ahead or 12 hours back. Then, to make a connection at Kennedy Airport for your overseas flight, you merely come in the night before, enjoy a lovely dinner out, a Broadway show, or a visit with relatives or friends, and then have a good night's sleep. The flight, instead of leaving at 9:00 P.M. departs at *9:00 A.M.* It is just past breakfast time for you.

Meantime, in London it is 2:00 P.M. Everyone there has finished lunch and has gone back to work. On this particular day, to make your journey even more enjoyable, the weather calls for sunshine and warm temperatures. You board your plane, fly five tiring hours, eating the same airline food (or a reasonable facsimile thereof), seeing the same movie next to the same seat companion, who still crosses over your legs every 20 minutes to make his/her way to the lavatory, and you arrive in London at 2:00 P.M. eastern standard time, which is 7:00 P.M. local time. Londoners are about to have their dinner. Their body clocks somehow seem closer to yours. You clear Customs, less bleary-eyed than you felt on the overnight flight, and make your way to your hotel, arriving about 8:00 or 9:00 P.M. their time, which is 3:00 or 4:00 P.M. your time. You unpack, eat lightly, and go to sleep after a hot bath; when you awaken in the morning, you will be much closer to "real time" than you would have been on the other trip.

SOME TIPS TO MINIMIZE JET LAG

Of course, it is not quite that simple. Most flights from here to Europe depart at night, but day flights do exist. Shop for one. Even so, there will be travel problems and there will be jet lag. There will probably be the waking up at 5:00 A.M. filled with excitement. But I assure you that the trip will seem easier for you and the response of your body will just not seem as severe as it has been before. If it is impossible to travel the way I've suggested, there are other tips you might well heed:

• Try to depart well rested. I mentioned the bon voyage parties in an earlier chapter. It can decrease your jet lag if you avoid them altogether.

• On longer flights, try the stopover trick that I suggested previously. Stop for one day at a city along the way—one you've always wanted to see.

• Athletes try to arrive at distant destinations from four to five days before the event in which they are competing. For the traveler on a limited time schedule, this is usually impossible, but it does give you a good idea of just how important it is to begin your touring as well rested as you can be.

• On a short trip of just a few days' duration, try to keep your schedule as close to the one at home as possible. This is a trick used by flight attendants on international airlines, and it works beautifully for them. A dear friend of mine named Anita Quaranta used to fly for Alitalia Airlines, and I'd see her often when she flew to New York. After a while I noticed that she wore two watches, one set for New York time and the other still on Rome time, her home base. She followed the Rome clock in everything she did, and she used the New York clock only to tell her when it was time to be back at the airport again. Thus, when we had dinner, she would eat a light, early-morning breakfast. If I telephoned in midafternoon, I usually awakened her, for she was on her "sleep" time. The next night, when she returned to Rome, her body clock would arrive home still on its own time.

• For the vacation traveler, the flight-attendant trick is not realistic. The next best thing is to get your own body clock on the local time as quickly as possible.

• Sleep on the plane if you can, even if it's for just an hour or so. My suggestion about taking along eyeshades and earplugs will help (except for the seat companion who edges over your legs every 20 minutes).

• Make sure you exercise, or, at the very least, walk up and down the aisles of the plane from time to time. This keeps your body functions active. (You might take another look at Chapter 5.)

• Avoid heavy meals both before you leave and aboard the plane. (Of course, meals aboard planes have become skimpier and more inedible as the years go by, so this is an easy rule to follow.)

• The suggestion about meals should also be taken seriously on your arrival. Eat lightly for the first few days. I must admit that there are some countries that tempt me with their cooking, and eating lightly is a difficult resolution to keep. I try to avoid Italy's pasta and its luscious Monte Bianco dessert (a mound of chestnut purée covered with whipped cream)—at least for a few hours!

• Keep your alcohol consumption to a minimum while flying. Two drinks at an altitude of 5,000 feet can have the same effect as four drinks at sea level.

• Carbon monoxide increases your fatigue when you fly. Try to cut down on your smoking aboard the aircraft.

• Stay away from pills if at all possible. I am speaking of sleeping pills, tranquilizers, and any other pills that will affect the body functions. Since travel across many time zones already has a strong impact on the body, any additional negative influence can only increase the chances that your body clock will tell the wrong time for many more hours.

• When you arrive, take a warm bath as a part of your unpacking procedure.

• Take one easy day to rest up after your trip. If you must sightsee on the first day (and I fully understand the urgency to "be" a part of a new city), make sure that it's a light day with very little walking.

• Take a nap that first afternoon.

A WORD ABOUT DRUGS

I am not, by nature, a "pill taker." I resist medication until the last moment. I prefer to wait until warned by my doctor that I will no doubt be stricken by bubonic plague if I do not take my tablet; and when I finally do take my pill, it works on me like a charge of dynamite, possibly because my body is normally free of society's drug-solution to almost everything that ails us. Under normal travel conditions, I prefer to avoid the drugs that have been specially designed to help me sleep, help me travel, help me relax, or help me wake up. If I suffer from jet lag (and I do) I prefer to let nature take its own sweet course to bring my body back to the time zone in which I am temporarily living. But that is a personal view, and some would disagree.

This chapter would be less than complete if I did not report (however subjectively) the fact that there has been some experimental work done on drugs to ease the problems of jet lag. As yet, they are not fully tested. But if and when they finally go on the market as a regular medication for time-zone syndrome, I still do not think that I would personally recommend them. Nonetheless, the thinking behind this experimenting is fascinating.

It stands to reason that if the body clock speeds up (short days and short nights) on the eastbound journey, the proper drug would slow it down. To that end, researchers have been experimenting with lithium carbonate, a drug that tends to retard the functions of the body. My research also tells me that this is the same drug given to manic depressives, leading a coward like me to assume that my personality will promptly change if I should dare try the drug. (Of course, some of my fellow workers have suggested anonymously that it might change my personality for the *better*, but I have ignored them.)

Going westbound, the body clock slows down—the days and nights are longer. A trip from New York to California, for example, can easily be made in full daylight, with departure at 9:00 A.M. from the East Coast and arrival before lunch in Los Angeles. The day has stretched for the passenger. A drug called imipramine hydrochloride, which speeds up the body clock, has been used by pilots with some success.

Frankly, I prefer to suffer my mild cases of jet lag and put it all down to the joys of travel and the small price we pay for living in a jet age. There is nothing we can really do to eliminate it, but we can certainly try to alleviate its effects. There have been hundreds of articles written about it in airline magazines, in travel literature, and in the newspapers. No one has yet found a way to avoid it except by staying at home—and I, for one, will never accept that solution.

As I said before, we do the best we can. And somehow it all works out. We adjust, each of us, differently, and in a different span of time—but adjust we do. All too soon you will be in familiar surroundings, sorry that the trip is over but glad to be back to your house and your job and your neighbors. And through it all you will be aware of one thing—a fresh case of jet lag. It is dinnertime when you get home, but you feel that instead of roast chicken, you must have orange juice, toast, eggs, and coffee! You have, without doubt, left your body clock over there!

INTERLUDE: SOME REMINISCENCES

When I reread what I have written about motion sickness and jet lag and airport problems and the thousand and three things that can go wrong—and sometimes do—I begin to feel that, somewhere in all the words and all the warnings, the real meaning of my travel will somehow be lost. It would be sad if that were the end result. So, give me a moment to pause, a moment to reflect, a moment to think.

Travel is very much like the rest of life. After the trip is over, we somehow manage to forget the pain and to remember only the good things. My father fought for three years in World War I and was severely wounded three times; yet the only stories I remember him recounting when I was a child were those of fun and joy and camaraderie. It was not until I questioned him in later years that he thought long and deeply and shared with me the agony of the times.

And so with travel. I can remember the most horrendous flights, the most difficult times in jungles of Asia, the most frightening experiences, if I care to think about them. And yet, these have become the funny stories of today, the regaling of friends with laughter and colorful descriptions of how we were arrested in Cambodia for what turned out to be a misunderstanding.

It was not funny when it happened—it was uproarious once we returned home.

We forget the jet lag, we forget the rudeness we encountered in a particular restaurant, we forget the bout with Montezuma's Revenge—or, at least, the immediate discomfort and pain are long since gone. The photographs we bring back are those of temples, shots of us and our companions that were taken much too far away to make out any detail, a lovely still of our guide in the jungle with his head cut out of the frame of the picture, and two hundred slides of the same sunset taken from the hotel balcony. And, at the least provocation, we will haul them out and happily show them to any and all who happen to be in the vicinity. But there are no slides of the problems.

On the long trip to Australia that I wrote of earlier in the book, I frankly cannot remember all my feelings of tiredness or jet lag. What I do remember most is flying over Australia at dawn, having just taken off from Darwin on the last leg to Sydney. The sun was still below the horizon, and suddenly, as I opened my sleepy eyes, the entire sky turned *green!* I had never seen a green sunrise before—I have not seen one since; but it stays with me to this day, a full 20 years later.

I can remember my first trip to Rome, a city I had never seen though I had lived in Europe right after World War II. We were there to do a TV fashion special for NBC, and my "New York head" as well as my New York body clock came right along with me. Things had to be done, locations scouted, crews rounded up, cables sent, models hired, meetings held, and scripts discussed with the stars, Celeste Holm and Domenico Medugno. There were at least a thousand complex things that had to be taken care of before the show could be taped. The pace was so fast when we arrived that I just forgot where I was—I could easily have been doing the show in Jersey City. Rome lay outside, waiting.

I underestimated my Italian friends, though. It was they who taught me a lesson. That first day in Rome, I spent the time scouting 22 locations, and we grabbed a 15-minute lunch at an outdoor counter. The pace was so rapid that, when I think of it, I am reminded today of a wonderful cartoon in the *New Yorker* magazine some years ago. A harried woman tourist rushes up to the entrance of the Louvre and shouts to the guard, "Where's the Mona Lisa? Hurry up—I'm double parked!" Such was our pace on the first day. The second day, they talked me into doing only ten locations, and we took one hour for lunch. By the third day, my clock finally slowed to Roman time and I scouted three locations in the morning, then joined my friends, my clients, and my crew for a *four-hour* repast.

And what a lunch it was! We were in Tivoli, near Hadrian's Villa, and we all sat on the terrace of a restaurant that was located right beneath the ruins of the Temple of Diana. The sun was shining, the Roman pines surrounded us, the carafes of wine kept coming; the joy and the incandescence of the moment can still be felt when I write now, and I find that I am smiling as I recall that lunch.

The final touch was a gift from my Italian friends. I am commonly known as a "dessert freak" and, there in the sunlight, after the wine, after the delicious veal and the tender, baby greens of the spring salad, the waiter came out bearing a large, overflowing, glistening lemon soufflé—and it was all mine, every last morsel of it. When the lunch was over, there was no sense going out to check another location—my Roman friends had won. My clock began to tick more slowly. It mattered not—the show was bound to be a success, for we had all fallen in love with the city. We apparently then communicated our feelings to the television audience, for one of the New York reviews later said, ". . . forget the fashions—we're taking the first plane to Rome!"

Think back, then, to your own trips. Think back to the little things you remember that made the trip memorable—the tiny cafe in the tiny street in the tiny village, the merchant you met while shopping for souvenirs, the sunlight and warmth on the isolated beach edging a cove of green water. You may even have forgotten that the enchanting little cottage you stayed in had huge mosquitoes buzzing around your head while you tried to sleep. For often hidden in the worst of times are some of the best of times!

All of my travel life I have been hearing the statement, "You should have been here last week (or next week). This is just the wrong time of the year." Or possibly it rains during the sunny season and no one can understand why. If I had only been there last week, when the sun was shining brightly . . . .

But I do remember being in one place just at the proper moment—an accident of time and space, to be sure. We were traveling in Cambodia near Angkor Wat. It has since become a sad and desolate land, but those were the times when the temples were open to the visitor who came from Bangkok via a DC-3 and landed on a strip carved out of the rice paddies. On the third day of working in the jungles around Siem Reap, we found ourselves deep in the forest. As we came around a bend, there before us was the huge head of an ancient Khmer statue, and out of the head grew a sensuous, twisting tree, its roots firmly planted in the stone. The roots looked like a piece of runny cheese (it was, in fact, called a "fromage tree"). The incredible thing about the scene was that the sun came through the trees and illuminated the entire statue in a shaft of brilliant light. Suddenly, through the forest came a Land-Rover bearing a British photographer, who leaped out and shouted to us as he clicked away with his camera, "You're in luck—this is the only hour of the only day of the year that the sun shines on that statue!" Finally, we had made it. We were somewhere at the right time!

Again—with an experience like that, we barely remember that it was also on that trip that we were arrested by the Cambodian National Police, a trip on which we had terrible supply problems, food problems, and airline problems. All that remains is a glow and a sense of loss when we read of Cambodia today.

I will not bore you with all my travel tales. You are welcome to view my own out-of-focus slides while I delight you with stories of my trip to Vietnam where my hosts served French lamb, thinking that I would not like Vietnamese cooking—and all the while, I had been an amateur aficionado of the cuisine, anxious to arrive there so that I could taste the famous Vietnamese crab dishes. Or I will tell about the row upon row of colorful saris I planned to shoot as they lay drying in the sun on the beach off Bombay—forgetting that it was monsoon season. And that reminds me for an instant of the Italian farmer who gave us a gift of peaches and grapes when we unknowingly trespassed on his property. I also recall buying a fresh fish from the fishermen on the Caspian Sea in Iran and bringing it back to the hotel to be cooked. The chef promptly ruined it and we ended up eating a spare can of sardines that we had been carrying for three weeks. A thousand memories, and we each carry our own.

But while this interlude lets me reminisce about my own joyous travel life, this book is dedicated to making each of *your* trips easier and more enjoyable. I merely want to pass on the advice and experiences that will help to make it so.

Now, back to the business of the book. What has preceded and what will follow can ease the fleeting discomforts of travel, while helping you bring back only the happiest recollections.

8

"GESUNDHEIT"— THE COMMON COLD AND OTHER MINOR FLYING PROBLEMS

With Some Thoughts on How to Deal with Them— and with Special Consideration for the Fearful Flyer...

Some of us have a superb sense of bad timing. Whether it is instinctive, physical or emotional, psychosomatic, or truly the result of some unforeseen circumstance, we are, purely and simply, victims of fate. Throughout our lives, minor catastrophes haunt us just as we are about to embark on some important phase of our lives. When I was a teenager, my face broke out in pimples just before the senior prom, to which I was to escort the love of my young life, after pursuing her for most of the previous semester.

Some of us manage to get a severe case of stomach upset right before an important dinner party, others of us spill ketchup on our trouser legs right before an important meeting. As a matter of fact, on a recent business trip, I wore my best suit, and took no extra clothing because I was only to be in

Chicago overnight and then return home. The flight was particularly bumpy and the flight attendants had a difficult time in maneuvering through the plane. I was sitting in my usual aisle seat and managed to have various and sundry foods and liquids spilled on me by the flight attendants *four separate times* on the same trip! For those of you interested in excruciating details, I arrived in Chicago with a small spot of coffee on my knee, the remains of orange juice on my jacket pocket, stains from a half-empty plate of canneloni on the other leg, and salad dressing on my shirt collar. The first time I was annoyed, the second time moderately angry, the third time I threatened to sue the airline, and by the fourth disaster I laughed. The flight crew presented me with a free airline coupon good for *four* dry cleanings at their expense. I could not bear to cash it in. I keep it in my office as a souvenir.

Of course, there are times when a bad sense of timing can turn out to be a distinct advantage. It worked well for me during World War II when I was hospitalized at training camp with pneumonia, and I complained and moaned and cried out at the injustice of it all. While I was thus inactive, my battalion was shipped overseas to land on the Normandy beaches on D-Day. So if you are a victim of bad timing in life, as I am, always remember that it can't be helped and it might just work out for the best.

Which brings me to the reason for all this discussion in the first place. You are about to embark on a long-awaited trip. Two days before you depart, you catch a cold—not just an ordinary, run-of-the-mill, garden variety cold, but a real humdinger. Possibly you have gone outside with a wet head after shampooing, and my mother would then tell you that God is punishing you. The reason is not important. You are going to board an airplane and you are, no doubt, going to be miserable.

It is, considering the state of the world, a minor problem and it is not enough to postpone or delay your trip. Nevertheless, it will make life even more uncomfortable for those few hours of flying, and there are ways to ease the trip and make your journey more bearable. This is also true for those who suffer from earaches or inner ear problems, for the flyers who have just been to the dentist or are having other work done on their teeth, and for those who are fearful of even getting aboard anything that leaves the ground and goes soaring into the stratosphere.

THE COMMON COLD AND THE NOT-SO-COMMON ONES

You have one advantage in this instance. You know beforehand that you have the cold and that you are going to fly with it, whether you like it or not. So if this should happen, here are some tips that will help minimize your distress:

• Carry a nasal decongestant with you in your pocket or purse.

• An antihistamine will also help in relieving the symptoms. Use it whenever you feel discomfort, but keep in mind that the worst period will be during descent, when the pressure changes rapidly. So make certain that you treat yourself about one hour before the plane is due to take off, and again as you feel the aircraft dip for its descent to the airport. Most modern jets are programed for about a 30-minute descent from flying altitude to landing.

• Try not to drink wine during your flight. For people such as I, who love wine with lunch or dinner, this can be another hardship, but wine has a tendency to intensify the feeling of congestion in the nose and sinus passages.

• When flying with a cold, you may be particularly susceptible to changes of altitude and cabin pressurization. Suck on some cough drops or hard candies. Chew gum (even if you were told that it's not polite). Anything that will relieve the pressure on the ears will help, even a series of good, solid yawns or swallows.

ADJUSTING TO PRESSURE

You may have noticed, as I have, that as the plane starts to dip into its descent, the babies aboard begin to cry loudly. Of course, they may have been crying loudly all through the trip, as many do, but there is a special howl of pain that we experienced travelers can distinguish from the usual cry that only means no one is paying attention to them. Babies seem to be sensitive to changes of cabin pressure, even more sensitive than adults. As a result, their ears clog and they feel uncomfortable. And so do we.

During the early days of jet travel, planes were not pressurized as well as they are today, and many of us who flew often were subject to severe bouts of ear pain and inner ear infection. It is not so common today, but every once in a while you will notice that your ears clog and your hearing, as a result, almost disappears. There are several ways to handle this problem. The easiest is to yawn or swallow deeply, just as I suggested for ear problems due to a cold. The second way is to hold your nose tightly with your fingers and then blow hard, keeping your mouth firmly shut. Either way, the purpose is to put enough pressure between your inner ear and mouth to enable the passage to open. When you're successful, you will feel a strong "pop" and your hearing will return. You can also expect a sharp, short pain in the ears as the passage opens.

In any case, this is another of those minor phenomena that happen most frequently when the plane is on its final descent. In my own experience with this pressure problem, I've sometimes found that if I clear the passage once while aboard, it does not recur again on that flight. On other trips, I have been victim several times during the journey. I can remember one case in which it lasted for about two hours after I disembarked. Overall, though, it happens very seldom to most of us. It is not a serious problem unless you are flying with an inner ear infection, in which case your doctor should be consulted before you leave.

DENTAL PROBLEMS

The best advice I can give here is to have all your dental work done well before you plan to take your trip. There are two very good reasons:

• It is the easiest way to avoid tooth pain during flight.

• Dental work done in most parts of the world is absolutely horrendous. I will probably have my visas lifted by unfriendly countries for saying this, but you do *not* want to be a dental emergency in most countries. It's the kind of thing that can ruin your trip, and your teeth.

So, along with planning your intinerary and getting your shots, make sure you have your dental work done far enough in advance so that you do not board the plane right after surgery. If you've had root canal work or a tooth extracted, there may be a small air pocket in the gum or near the teeth, and the change in pressure in the plane will, in turn, exert still more pressure on that pocket. The result can range from mild discomfort to severe pain.

There have been times, however, when I've had to visit my dentist a day or so before a trip, mostly because, frequently, I am not certain just when I will have to leave. And, for the tourist, there also may just be a time when a dental emergency occurs and you certainly don't want to postpone the trip which you've been counting on for so long. Of course you should depart on schedule, but make certain that your dentist gives you some kind of pain killer to take with you. Keep it in your flight bag or right on your person in case you need it.

In these rare instances, I have also asked my dentist if he might recommend the name of a capable person at my destination who would be able to see me should I need help. Dentists are like filmmakers. Just as I know the names of many talented documentarians around the world, I have found that my dentist and periodontist have friends in their profession ranging from Brazil to Ghana. If you don't have a name, Chapter 20, on medical emergencies, may be of help to you.

ALLERGY TO INSECTICIDES

I remember my first trip to Asia—landing, and the feeling of excitement at finally getting there. But we were not allowed to disembark. The plane got hotter and stuffier by the moment, the door finally opened, and someone in a white uniform with epaulets walked through the plane spraying some kind of foul-smelling insecticide. There are still many places in the world where this is done as a matter of routine in order to avoid importing unwanted insects. Many travelers who are allergic to ragweed may also be affected by these sprays, for the pyrethrum insecticides are, in fact, extracted from a plant that is quite similar to ragweed.

If you are one of those who is allergic, and you are traveling to any tropical area where such spraying may take place:

- Ask the flight attendant if the plane will be sprayed at your destination.

- If it will, ask for a wet towel before landing. When the Health Officer comes aboard with the spray can, breathe through the wet towel.

- Continue to breathe through the towel for at least five minutes after the spraying, to allow the insecticide to settle.

THE "WHITE KNUCKLE" FLYER

I mentioned earlier that I was a "white knuckle" flyer for many of my first years of flying. (The term, of course, comes from the color of your knuckles when you tightly grasp the seat arms in fear and trepidation.) Every time the plane lurched or bumped, I was convinced that we would turn upside down. My life would pass in front of me in full color before each takeoff and landing. After all, how can anything that heavy even get off the ground, let alone fly at thirty-five thousand feet where the air is so thin anyway.

If it will help at all, I must say that the constant travel, the millions of miles, the repeated experiences of turbulence, of taking off and landing, of just becoming familiar with planes and airports and procedures, will eventually minimize or completely eradicate any fears of flying that you may have. It worked with me. I now read, sleep, think, and concentrate while on a plane. In fact, I even *look forward* to my flights, for they are the only times of peace and quiet when there are no telephones ringing, no urgent calls that must be taken care of right away. Too, I have learned much about planes over these years; I know about their sophisticated backup systems, and I believe that I am safer in one of them than I am on the ground with a New York taxicab driver who is taking me from the airport to my home. I remember, with a smile, the final announcement of a pilot on one of my flights: "Ladies and gentlemen, in a few moments, we will be landing at John F. Kennedy Airport in New York. The safest part of your journey is now over. Please be careful driving."

Of course, I have convinced no one. Those of you who are the fearful flyers will read my words with a strong sense of being lied to, and with a knot in your stomach. In addition, not everyone flies as much as I do, and taking one or two trips a year is not enough to remove the fear of entering an aircraft. It was once my own feeling as well. And there are members of my family who will not get aboard one of those things, who carry with them a continued frustration that they would, indeed, like to see the world, but not if they have to fly.

There are programs that have been developed especially for the passenger who is afraid of flying. A very popular one has been created by some of the pilots of Pan American, on their own, and without the official involvement of the airlines. It is now available all over the country and it's called "Fearful Flyers." The program consists of a gradual acclimatization, and the results have been quite good. If you're interested, write to Fearful Flyers, c/o Pan American World Airways, Room 4523, Pan Am Building, New York, NY 10017.

One of my friends reports a less scientific but just as reliable approach. Some of you may also have been witness to this method while you have been aboard a plane during takeoff. He writes in his last letter to me: ". . . sitting next to me was an Ecuadorian woman who kept wildly crossing herself during our takeoff. It worked. The plane took off."

90

9

GOD'S COUNTRY AIN'T LIKE THE TRAVEL ADS SHOW US

... Women (Pregnant) Traveling with Child, Traveling with Children, Children Traveling Alone, Traveling with Pets ...

I love to read the travel section of the Sunday newspaper. Not only do I mentally visit the places to which I've not yet been, but the letters from readers give me new ideas, new tips about travel, and sometimes I can relive through them the joy I've had in some foreign place, as well as sympathizing with some of the problems they met along the way. But, in reading the weekly stories about traveling to Dallas or Dakar, Peoria or Paris, Cairo-Illinois (pronounced Cay-ro) or Cairo-Egypt (pronounced Ky-ro), I also make it a point to look at the advertising that fills the pages. Ah, the promises of pleasure, the heralding of excitement and pampering and love! But when I look closely at the photographs that accompany these semifictional promotions, I realize that those people are not *me!* As a matter of fact, they are not mostly *you,* either.

Except for some photographs that depict idyllic, retouched views of our destinations (sunsets, hotel rooms, golf courses, swimming pools, or totally empty beaches), almost every travel ad today presents the resort, the trip, the cruise, the flight in terms of a young, heterosexual couple—he dark and handsome and intense (with a sort of a vapid "model's " look), she generally in a bikini or some other revealing outfit, both of them in their early thirties. This is a very important thing to notice—they are always in their early thirties. By their gestures and their looks alone, you know that this irresistible vacation is being spent by two equally irresistible people.

IS THE FANTASY THE REALITY?

Last Sunday, I dug out the travel section of the newspaper from under a pile of unread magazines and I went through it, page by page, to see if my observations were correct. Before me, as I write, I have a selected collection of clippings that I've cut from just one issue:

• "Just the Two of Us" it reads, she lying at the water's edge, her arm draped around his darkly sensual neck, her tiny bathing suit revealing just enough.

• Another young couple stand at the tennis net, but their look is exactly the same as the one worn on the faces of the people who were at the water's edge.

• One ad has a couple (why do they all look alike?) standing together on a sailboat near a Greek city that lazily appears out of the mist at their backs, and six other ads show couples (backlit by sun) walking hand in hand on a pure, untouched beach, or coming out of the placid, waveless water.

• Aha! A woman alone—except on closer inspection, the woman (in a bikini) is being pursued by Prometheus, who has just come out of the water in the distance.

• One ad, indeed, does show a woman lifting *a baby* into the air, glad that she took her child along. But it is placed very carefully next to three photos showing our young couple dancing, our young couple on motorbikes, and our same young couple playing tennis. Another ad shows the chef aboard our ship displaying a typical lunch of caviar and lobster. But here again, they have been careful to include photographs of couples—on deck, on sailboats, in the lounges.

Is this the fantasy in which we really see ourselves? Only young, beautiful, sexual, carefree, and obviously wealthy? Where are the older folks, such as the author ("older," according to the advertising agencies, being defined as anyone over 35)? Where are the people traveling with children, the woman or the man alone, the woman traveling with a woman, the man traveling with a man, the traveler with some physical problems, or those of us who don't look quite so good in a bathing suit or a bikini? Don't we travel, too? Or do *we* also think of ourselves only as we see the models in the advertisements? I must mention that there is one ad that runs week after week in our Sunday travel section, and I have fallen madly in love with a dark, long-haired young woman who wears a white, revealing bikini while being held tenderly by the usual dark escort. I am so taken with her, in fact, that I do not even know what resort she is advertising!

My Italian friends taught me a saying: "The fantasy is the reality." Maybe it is, but most of the people I've seen on my trips just don't look like the ads. However, if you do resemble the people I've described above, you can skip this chapter and move on. For the rest of us, here are some suggestions that might help make your trip easier, should you fit any of the categories that follow.

IF YOU'RE PREGNANT

Of course, you understand that this is one area in which I cannot speak from experience. Nevertheless, my travel files are rich with articles and books filled with advice for just this situation.

First of all, it stands to reason that your doctor will know about your forthcoming trip abroad, and you will have discussed your needs and the possible emergencies that might arise, all of them depending upon the month of term and your reaction to the pregnancy.

If you are going to a country where sanitation or general health conditions may be hazardous, send for the booklet mentioned earlier: *Health Information for International Travel* (U.S. Department of Health, Education and Welfare, Public Health Service, Center for Disease Control, Atlanta, GA 30333). It is one of the few guides I've seen that specifically indicates immunization and contraindications for pregnant women. As a matter of fact, if your trip will require *any type* of immunization, you might want to read the book, for it covers the precautions to be taken during pregnancy for a range of potential diseases: cholera, yellow fever, malaria, measles, and rubella.

Remember, the vaccines given to the traveler who is pregnant will probably not affect the adult, but precautions are generally taken because of the fetus. Remember, too, that live virus vaccines are generally not given to pregnant women for just that reason, so it's a good idea to know exactly what the potential health problems are in the area to which you're traveling. For example, live measles vaccines would probably not be given to you. In areas that still have malaria, your doctor will probably suggest that you take chloroquine, while other drugs such as pyrimethamine would not be recommended because their effects on pregnant women are not known.

Essentially, there is no reason that you cannot travel while pregnant, all other things being equal. But you might just take note of some of these added tips:

• Of course, see your doctor. You are basically subject to the same travel problems that any international traveler might encounter, with a few added considerations.

• If you have additional questions or if you are traveling to an area not generally covered by available health information, get the booklet suggested above; also, ask your explicit questions at the consulate or embassy of the country to which you are traveling.

• Keep in mind that travel by air in late pregnancy may well precipitate labor. An occasional child has, indeed, been born aboard a plane. If you are in your ninth month of pregnancy, the airline may request that you present a certificate from your doctor approving your travel and giving the approximate expected date of birth.

• Make sure you are prepared with advice about doctors, hospitals, and emergency care at your destination. See Chapter 20 if your doctor cannot give you the information you need.

• If you are close to term, make certain that you check with the local medical contact upon your arrival. There are times that you might come armed with the name and address of a local doctor only to find that he has been transferred, the phone is out of order, or the information is incorrect. Recently, on a trip to a small village in Ecuador, we found that the doctor whose name had been given to us had been transferred six months before and news had not yet reached the capital city of Quito!

• If you do not have the name of a local doctor or hospital, check in with the American or Canadian consulate or embassy and make note of the information you receive from them. They generally have the names and numbers of available medical help.

By following these small, common sense tips, there is no reason at all that you should not enjoy your trip. In addition, there is one other minor area of satisfaction that should make you smile; it involves the only fare structure not covered in the airline rate sheets: Just think about it—two (or more) of you are traveling for the price of one!

TRAVELING WITH CHILDREN

The plane had just taken off from Fiumicino Airport in Rome and I settled back for what I thought was to be a long, pleasant flight to New York—time to read and to sleep and to remember. But the No Smoking sign had no sooner gone off than the trip began in hysteria as a woman's voice shrieked, "Steven, sit down and put your seat belt on!" And a few moments later, "Steven, sit *down*—if you don't sit down I'll smack you!"

Needless to say, for almost 11 hours, the voice echoed through the cabin while Steven ran up and down the aisles, made life miserable for 130 passengers, and gave his ineffectual mother a case of hypertension. To this day, when I see a child running up and down the aisles, I mutter to myself, "Steven, put your seat belt on!" It obviously affected me more than I care to admit.

Children do travel today, and they are taken on trips more than ever before. Many will grow up completely acclimated to airplanes and long journeys. I have friends who have been taking their 13-year-old daughter to Europe with them since she was 5 years old. The cars on our highways are filled with children on their way to Yellowstone or to visit grandma, and the ships have begun to make special arrangements for infants, for toddlers, and for the more active older child who is taken along on vacation. There is no one general rule to follow, for all children are different and all needs are personal and individual. After all, even while Steven was running rampant up the aisle of the plane, there were five other kids playing quietly or sleeping. The important thing is to plan carefully—from packing to arrival. Among the tips that follow, you may very well find the one that will be the solution to having your child travel right with you as a good companion rather than a "Steven-put-your-seat-belt-on."

FLYING WITH THE VERY YOUNG

We were leaving Dublin on the morning flight. It was right before Christmas and the plane was to be filled to capacity. In addition, the front end of the DC-8 was designed to hold cargo, which pushed everyone back into the rear section of the plane. I suppose I remember the flight most vividly because of the number of infants aboard. Every second passenger was carrying a baby—and all of them were on their way to New York to show off the newborn to the grandparents. There were, at my last hysterical count, 56 *squalling, sleeping, crying, squirming infants aboard!* If you should happen to get aboard a flight such as my Christmas one, most of the tips that follow will be of absolutely no value. Close your eyes, hold your breath, and hope that the trip seems short. However, on an ordinary flight, here are some things to keep in mind:

• The most important thing you can do is to let the carrier know about the baby at the time that you make your reservations.

• Wait at least a week before taking a newborn on that first flight. It takes that long for the tiny lungs to become stable.

• Before you leave home, pack a flight bag especially for the child. It should be made of plastic or some other water-resistant material, in case of spillage. Pack it with several bottles of formula, diapers, nipples, pins, powders, lotions, and anything else you might need on the flight. Most airlines will warm the bottles for you, but flight attendants are generally not allowed to mix the formulas.

• Keep in mind that airlines are subject to delays due to weather or mechanical problems. Make certain you have enough supplies to last a few extra hours in case your flight is delayed or cancelled.

• Dress the infant in clothes that are easy to undo, for you will have to change diapers right at the seat.

• Request a bulkhead seat (front of plane) and the airline will probably provide a portable bassinet that attaches right to the wall in front of you. However, most airlines require that you hold the child in your arms during takeoff and landing.

• Ask to preboard the plane. Again, most airlines are prepared for this and you will generally hear a preboarding announcement made for passengers traveling with small children.

• You are generally allowed to bring your own bassinet, provided that it can be securely fastened by the seat belt to an adjacent seat, and provided that you purchase a ticket for the child (usually half rate).

• If you use the folding type of umbrella stroller, you may want to take it aboard the plane with you rather than check it through to your final destination. For once you arrive at the other end, you may find it easier to carry your child in the stroller than in your arms.

• You may not bring an infant seat aboard the planes of many airlines. The Federal Aviation Administration states that these seats may be dangerous in an emergency and they are not approved for use on takeoff and landing. Basically, such seats are designed for automobiles rather than airplanes.

• Be prepared to do much of the work yourself. The flight attendants are busy during mealtime, and should there be more than one infant aboard, it is quite impossible for them to give more than a fleeting amount of help during those hectic times.

• Try to arrange to feed your infant during takeoff and landing, if possible. These are the times that the altitude changes affect them most, and sucking helps relieve the pressure and prevent earaches.

Overall, babies are generally excellent air travelers—they sleep most of the day, they are fed often and are thus not on the "body clock" syndrome of their parents, and the airlines have really worked at making life easier for the traveling family. If you do have special problems or special requests, contact the carrier on which you've booked your trip. Each of them varies with regard to the services they offer, with some international airlines providing brand-name baby foods, bottle warmers, and even a good supply of diapers. Agents are available at the airport to help you preboard and to assist you on the other side. Some airlines have gone so far as to publish little pamphlets that will help you make your first flight together easier and more pleasant. You can write to TWA, for example, for their free pamphlet, *Air Travel for Children.*

In terms of health, it is, of course, imperative that you get advice from your pediatrician before taking an infant on any extended journey, particularly if the area to which you're going may be dangerous to the baby's well-being. It would take another book to cover all the potential problems—and precautions to be taken—pertaining to climate, water purity, immunizations, and the thousand things that must be considered if an infant is to be relocated in this world of ours. An excellent summary is given, however, in the book I recommended in Chapter 3, *The Traveller's Health Guide* by Dr. Anthony C. Turner, the Senior Overseas Medical Officer of British Airways. I would also suggest you read Chapter 11 of his book *Don't Forget the Children* if you anticipate any special problems, or if you are headed for a developing area of the world and taking your family with you.

IF YOU ARE BREAST-FEEDING

We spent a good part of last year in the Sierras and in the jungles of South America, producing some films for the Ecuadorian Ministry of Health and the United Nations. One of the subjects was "Breast-feeding and Immunology," and it was a superb education for those of us who come from contemporary, urban, North American societies. There seems to be no doubt that a natural immunology is passed from mother to child when the infant is breast-fed. In fact, we see more and more young mothers going back to nature, even here in the United States and Canada. Those of you who may be traveling to a permanent overseas location with your family, especially to the tropics, may be interested to know that the breast-fed infant seems to have a better chance of avoiding severe onsets of diarrheal diseases. Of course, gastroenteritis may well occur no matter how the child is being fed, since there are many more factors involved in preventing it—such as sanitation and general, all-around hygiene. But studies seem to indicate that the breast-fed infant is less susceptible.

In the matter of vaccinations, however, your doctor may feel that breast-feeding may present other problems. It is wise to discuss your destination and length of stay with your physician or your local health department well in advance of your departure date.

Inactivated or killed vaccines create no special problems for either mother or infant. If a live vaccine is used—such as smallpox, yellow fever, or the oral poliomyelitis vaccine—there are very strong contraindications for pregnant women which I mentioned before, and some lesser ones for the mother who is breast-feeding, since live vaccines multiply within the mother's body. However, the U.S. Public Health Service states that most are not transmitted through mother's milk, and those that are have very little effect on the infant. Depending upon your health and the condition of your baby, your own doctor may have some very strong opinions of his own on the subject. Check into it carefully.

BABIES ABOARD SHIP

For most parents, the idea of taking a cruise ship represents the perfect escape from the kids. For others, and the number seems to be on the increase, taking the children is part of the fun. In addition, there may be other reasons that the infant has to be taken along—possibly you are returning from an overseas assignment and the family is being relocated. Certainly, if you decide to go by sea, the baby will accompany you.

Just as in flying with a child, taking a ship requires some preplanning, not the least of which is to contact the line to find out just what facilities are provided for the very young. The answers may range from "Children, what are *they?*" to information about a complete range of services, such as those aboard the QE-2. This ship provides cribs, has a nursery, a children's playroom, high chairs, and a baby-sitting service. Here are some things that you might keep in mind if you plan to take a young child with you aboard a ship:

- Baby food is generally available aboard ship, but if you use a special brand, make sure you check to see that they carry it, or bring a supply aboard with you.

- It is quite possible to have baby food warmed for you by the steward, but it will take time. Friends of mine who travel with their children suggest that you take a small electric plate warmer along.

- Most large ships have a drugstore aboard and they are generally well equipped to handle the young traveler—having diapers, lotions, oils, and so forth. Take a small extra supply for emergencies, however.

• Staterooms come with a shower or a bathtub, depending upon how much you've decided to pay for the trip. Keep it in mind when you book your room, for a shower may be impossible if you have to bathe the baby in your stateroom.

• Try to make your arrangements for baby-sitters, special needs, feeding schedules as soon as you board the ship. Also remember that your own dinner or lunch schedule should be planned to coincide comfortably with the eating times of the baby.

CHILDREN IN THE CAR

In some ways, taking young children on a car trip is the easiest way to travel—assuming that the journey is not an endless one, with days and hours to be filled with games, sight-seeing tricks, car sickness, eating at odd hours, and the general malaise that accompanies the long trip to the vacation resort. For the tiny ones, the back seat can act as bed, changing table, game room, and dining room. For older children, the manufacturers have developed some ingenious car seats that let the young passenger stay amused at eye level with the countryside.

One word of warning, however, about traveling with *all* children—be sure you have some restraining device in use when the car is in motion. Car seats, car shields, harnesses, and even the normal safety belt for older children are all effective devices to prevent serious injury in case of collision. I'm sure that you, as I, have driven the highways and watched children in passing cars crawling over the driver, the front seat, the dashboard, and out of the windows while the car is in motion. I shudder when I see it, for, in case of an accident, it is the children who are most violently thrown around the inside of the car.

FOR THE OLDER CHILDREN

You know your own children, of course, and you know whether they behave well or miserably on a family trip. You know about their favorite toys, their favorite games, and their peculiar habits. Possibly they have never been on a plane or a ship before, but for children who have begun to walk, travel is essentially one great adventure. For every child who travels badly, there are ten or more who take the trip in stride. Certainly, children get restless when they feel confined for a long period of time, and your planning should include a supply of favorite toys, reading matter, and puzzles. But if the trip is to be a long one, hand these out one at a time so that boredom doesn't set in an hour after departure.

If your journey is to be by plane, a few extra suggestions are worth bearing in mind:

- As with infants, you can usually be preboarded on a flight by merely telling the agent that you are traveling with children.

- Make certain that you pack a separate flight bag for the child, just as you do for yourself. Include extra clothing that you might need on the flight, and keep in mind that it sometimes gets chilly at the higher altitudes, even though the cabin heat and pressure are supposed to be constant. Take along a warm sweater and an extra pair of woolen socks. Here again, this is one of those things that slips our mind when it's 95°F back home and we're much too hot to think that we'll ever be cold again.

- Bring along some nonjunk food snacks for the children, or pack a food basket and share a picnic with the young traveler (see Chapter 13). Meals and snacks on today's flights offer very little selection to choose from, and frequently the galley runs out of the main dish of your choice right before they get to your seat. It happens to me all the time.

- If your child is on a special diet, notify the airline when you or your travel agent make the reservations.

Most airlines today also present children with some kind of "junior airperson wings" that can be worn proudly as a memento of the flight. TWA calls them Junior Crew Members, British Airways makes them members of the Junior Jet Club. Frankly, I have always been jealous that it is only the children who get the plastic wings. I would love to have them myself, but I'm reluctant to ask.

And, there is one final note about children. I suppose we forget too often that children are people—*little* people, to be sure, but people nonetheless. When we travel with them, they require their own wardrobes, their own suitcases, their own vaccinations, and their own passports. As for the latter, I would strongly suggest that you do *not* get the family passport that is offered by the Department of State. This is a document that carries the photographs and the vital statistics of every member of the family in one passport booklet. The problem is an obvious one. Though it may save you money initially, and though you think you plan to travel together forever, you cannot separate at any time when crossing a border; you must, indeed, be together at all times, just as your passport photo shows. In case of emergency or should you decide to travel separately for any reason, it pays to have individual passports for every member of the family, even the children.

THE UNACCOMPANIED CHILD

The flight from Milan to New York took somewhere near 11 hours, a long journey battling Atlantic head winds all the way. The little Italian boy sat quietly in his seat at the bulkhead, dressed in his best blue suit, his hair combed back neatly, a large name tag dangling from his pocket. By the end of the first hour, the flight attendants had fallen in love with him, and by midflight every passenger had visited him to comment and speak to him, though he spoke no English at all. He was alone, he was on his way to visit his grandmother in the United States, and he was the airline's single, best, most loved passenger. His mother and father would have been proud of him.

Finally, the DC-8 began its long descent into Kennedy Airport and the weariness of the flight began to be replaced with anticipation. We all quite forgot about our young passenger sitting in front. The plane touched down, rolled to a slow stop, and the child began to cry. Through the cabin, his loud, plaintive wails shattered the hum of the idling engines, and the flight attendants rushed to see if they could help him. It turned out that nothing serious was wrong—it was just that, with all that attention from crew and from passengers, during the entire 11 hours no one had bothered to ask the youngster if he wanted to go to the bathroom, and he was just venting his frustration and the pain of his bladder.

I often smile when I see children who travel alone these days. They are, just as our little Italian passenger, mostly quiet, mostly well behaved—and all of them are pampered by passengers and airline personnel alike. There are certain children who must travel unaccompanied, and the anxious parents or relatives who leave them at the gate when they board the plane can generally rest assured that the airlines are quite capable of taking care of their small charges. It is done all the time. However, note that:

- Most airlines have an age minimum below which a child cannot travel alone. Usually, the age is five—and if he or she is younger, an escort or some responsible person must go along on the trip.

- A complete information sheet must be filled out so that the airline knows the name of the person meeting the child, telephone numbers for emergency, and your own name, address, and telephone number where you can be reached if necessary.

- If a flight is rerouted or delayed, the child will receive the same meals, hotel rooms, transportation, and other help given to all passengers, but additional fees—such as for baby-sitters or guardians—will be passed on to you.

Though the child is technically traveling "alone," you'll find that the airlines and their personnel are quite attentive. The child is escorted from the plane at the destination, generally after everyone else has disembarked. At that time, the person meeting the child or an airline agent will take charge.

And—one additional point to set your mind at ease—the little Italian boy was an exceptional story. Most children are asked whether they'd like to go to the bathroom. The rest of them have no qualms about letting the flight attendants know their needs!

TRAVELING WITH PETS

Over these wonderful years of being a producer and director in television and film, I've worked with many of the industry's extraordinary people. Of course, I have also worked with some of the industry's most miserable, spoiled, temperamental, unstable, childish, and untalented professionals, in spite of what their press agents write about them. I tend quickly to forget the latter.

Among the greats—and still a friend of mine today—is Celeste Holm. She and I have done many shows and films together, both here and abroad, and whenever she showed up on location, whether in Rome or Chicago, she was accompanied by her black and white, one-eyed miniature poodle, Maestro. The crews became so fond of the little dog that they finally gave Maestro his own director's chair, with his name painted across the back.

Of course, it is not unusual today to take your pet along on a trip, though

103

dogs seem to bear up under car trips better than cats do (ours, at least). We are, most of us, used to the needs of the pet as well as the special equipment necessary for traveling from here to there while hauling an animal along with us. It is a fact of life that *all* travel with pets will need advance planning, but I would like to speak more specifically at this point about international travel, first, and then cover some domestic tips that might help you on your trip.

Though Celeste took Maestro with her whenever she could, she found that international travel limited her options. One day she told me that she had cancelled a tour through Australia because of the quarantine regulations for the dog. There just was no way to take him along. In Australia, dogs and cats are listed under "illegal imports" and the rules for entry are these:

- The animal can be quarantined in Hawaii or in the United Kingdom before being shipped to Australia.

- If quarantine is in Hawaii, the length of time is six months' isolation, followed by a stay at the Brisbane Animal Station in Australia for a period of nine additional months!

- If quarantine is in the United Kingdom, then the animal must have at least six months' residence in Great Britain, followed by six months' quarantine there, followed by 60 days' quarantine in Australia if the dog or cat arrives by sea, and 90 days if it arrives by air.

For the vacationing traveler, this usually presents no problem; chances are that you will not take your dog or cat with you on a three-week airplane trip to any vacation spot. But if you were changing jobs and relocating, then you can begin to see why it's important to check with the consulate or your travel agent a long time in advance.

Certainly, not all countries are as severe as the example given above. Let's compare two that lie across the channel from one another and you'll see what I mean.

Great Britain. The dog or cat must be in quarantine for six months in a specially designated kennel. There are no exceptions, and the law is very strictly enforced with heavy penalties for violations.

France. You merely receive a certificate of good health from your local veterinarian in the United States or Canada. The certificate will be checked and the animal inspected upon arrival in France.

You can see that there is a vast difference in rules and regulations all over the world. You merely have a lot of homework to do before you depart. But then, I've said that before, haven't I? Incidentally, in Chapter 26 I've outlined the Customs regulations for bringing your pets back into the United States, and I've included some rules that govern the animals you might acquire on your trip abroad. After all, you never know when you might fall in love with an African elephant!

Domestically, the regulations may be easier, but the dog or cat can present some problems, depending upon its travel personality. We once owned a German shepherd (not the same one who was stung by the bee and who cut his paw all on one trip), and the mere sight of the back seat of a car gave him a severe case of motion sickness. Some animals have to be tranquilized, others take the trip easily and with aplomb. I'm sure that every pet owner could write a book about the animal that lives in his or her family.

- Domestic airlines will accept your pet, though with varying regulations. Some will allow small pets to travel in the cabin, so long as they are boxed. All of them require crating of some sort, and these are available for rental directly from the carrier. Large animals are carried in a specially pressurized baggage compartment.

- Dogs and cats can be taken on train trips, so long as they are in well-ventilated crates and so long as there is baggage service on the train. If you don't have your own carrier, check with the railroad. Amtrak has pet carriers available at major stations along their routes.

- If you are traveling by bus, you will have to send your pet on ahead by some other means of transportation, since interstate buses are not allowed to carry animals.

- The rules at hotels and motels vary. North Carolina, for example, has a state law that forbids pets from spending the night at any hotel or motel. For years, we spent our Chicago trips at the Edgewater Beach Hotel because it was the only place in town that accepted our dogs. When they tore it down, our hearts went with it. Make sure you check ahead to see if your pet is welcome at the lodging of your choice. Gaines Dog Food publishes a handy pamphlet listing accommodations that will accept your pet. It's called *Touring with Towser,* and it costs one dollar. Send to: Gaines *Touring with Towser,* P.O. Box 1007, Kankakee, IL 60901. It will take about four weeks.

And, here are a few other suggestions to help make the travel life of your pet more comfortable:

- Visit your vet before the trip and get some sedation for the animal if experience has shown you that your dog or cat will require it. Also get a certificate or tag of rabies vaccination to take along. Though some states technically require that you have one with you, we have never been asked for it. However, should your animal accidentally bite or scratch a child, you'll be required to provide it immediately.

- I suppose that the thing that most drives me slightly out of my mind is walking down a hot city street in the middle of summer and seeing an animal that has been left alone in a car, the windows closed and the sun beating down on a black, heat-absorbing top. The animal can suffer heat prostration or stroke; even slightly opening the windows is not enough to cool the car. If you can, take the animal with you if you must leave the car for any length of time.

- Cats are better travelers when they're placed in a carrier and then on the floor of the car. The scenery, moving by at 55 miles an hour (if you're obeying the speed limit) can terrify the poor animal. If the trip is a long one, think about shipping your cat by air.

On my trips by car, I have seen pet turtles, lemurs, rabbits, raccoons, hamsters, and snakes. I remember one trip on which we stopped at a turnpike restaurant and saw an eight year old walking on the lawn exercising her pet rooster. For each and for all of these unusual-pet categories, I have no good travel advice. I'm sure you know more about it than I do.

10

"O SOLO MIO"— I AM TRAVELING ALONE

Some Words of Wisdom for the Single Traveler and for the Traveler on a Fixed Budget . . .

I do most of my traveling with film crews that number anywhere from three to six people, but I take many of my business trips alone. The essential location survey and research and scouting trips are frequently unaccompanied, and I generally come back with the same complaints, the happy and unhappy memories of any single traveler in this world so geared to couples and groups.

I was in St. Louis recently, alone; it was the twelfth stop of a 17-city publicity book tour. Tired, anxious for it to be over, I was ready for a quiet evening—dinner accompanied only by a small bottle of wine. I asked my friends to name the best restaurant in the city and the consensus pointed to an Italian place, elegant in its isolation in the worst section of downtown St. Louis. Somehow restaurants like these seem to draw the "in" crowds, an oasis of elegance in the midst of poverty. The limousines and brand new sedans pulled up, and the red-coated attendants whisked the cars off the street into a guarded parking lot, away from the hangers-on who loitered near the city bus station. I fully realize that all my friends will recognize this restaurant by the description I have given, and if the owner should object, I shall deny everything—even though only one place in St. Louis meets this description. Read on.

It was early; they took no reservations, but being used to New York dining hours I was convinced that I should be able to get a single table at six in the evening. I was wrong. They were packed. The bar was crowded, the two-level dining room filled to capacity. I walked to the maitre d' and he looked behind me to see how many of my friends might be following me. Seeing no one, he turned to me, his cool eye on my solitary figure. I asked how long the wait would be and he shrugged, shook his head, and said, "Oh, I imagine about an hour, or even an hour and a half . . . ."

Up to this point, the reader wonders why I became upset. After all, the conversation thus far said nothing beyond any normal restaurant dialogue. It was the next sentence that put the finishing touch to my disillusionment. Haughtily, icily, he added, ". . . but that's an awfully long time to wait when you're *alone,* isn't it?" Of course, I did not wait.

At a dinner party the other evening, I mentioned to a group of friends that I was writing this book. The first comment was "Tell them about the problems the single traveler has!" followed by, "Don't forget to write about *two women* traveling." There is no doubt in my mind that some of the most serious travel inequities occur when we are forced to travel alone—or when we decide that we really *want* to travel alone. Not the least of these injustices is the famous (or infamous) "singles supplement"—the additional charge levied on the person who does not want to share a room with a known or unknown companion. If you have traveled alone, you have read—as have I—the ads that state: "All charges double occupancy." Therefore, if you travel with someone, the cost of the trip may run only $400 per person (double occupancy), and if you travel as a single, the rate surcharge will bring your trip to about $600!

THE WORLD CHANGES
FOR THE SINGLE

I think it's important to notice one big change in this area of travel, however. The word "single" no longer connotes the young unmarried below the age of 35. Certainly, if you look closely at those ads I mentioned, you will find age limits on many of the singles weekends or singles cruises (usually that magic number again—35). But I have two widowed friends who travel either as singles or together as companions, and both are nearing 60. People who are divorced, separated, or just loners may want to travel alone. And how about business people—the men and the growing number of women who travel all over the world as part of the job? We are also "singles" by any definition you can give. Though business hotels and restaurants in the United States, particularly, are geared to handle us, you'd be surprised at how often we are given the worst room or are sneered at by some haughty maitre d', just as I was in St. Louis. Five or ten years ago, it was nearly impossible for a woman executive to travel without harassment, and for her to even enter a bar for a quiet after-dinner drink was considered an invitation to every macho male in the place. I remember that I was once returning from a trip to France about ten years ago and my wife drove to the airport to pick me up. It was August, hot and humid. The airport air conditioning had broken down in the terminal— only the cocktail lounge was cool. My plane was four hours late and they wouldn't even let my wife into the bar unescorted to have a soft drink! She had to pace the hot, stuffy reception area for all those hours. She has since learned not to come to the airport to pick me up on a crowded holiday. weekend.

Things have changed somewhat, though in many foreign countries they are exactly the same as they've always been—and they will probably remain so forever. But I have learned, from listening to other experienced travelers and from my own observations, that there is absolutely no reason on this lovely earth why the single traveler should not enjoy a trip as much as the couples do. And keep this in mind: Many couples go off into the sunset and have an absolutely *terrible* time—just listen to the needling, the spats, the arguments, the discontent when you sit alone in a restaurant and you happen to overhear the pair sitting at the next table. In my weaker moments alone, I have accepted an invitation from someone dining near me to join his table. Within five minutes, I found myself wishing that I were alone again, with my own thoughts, my observations, my glass of wine.

THE SINGLES TOURS

This is probably the easiest group to cover, for all kinds of travel arrangements are available for people who want to travel alone and are willing to join a group. The travel agents have reams of materials on "singles weekends" and "singles cruises" and trips for people who like to ski together, play tennis, meet a prospective lover or mate, or just be surrounded by people to give them more security. Generally, these groups are quite specific as to age, but there are hundreds of trips available for all ages on luxury liners, by air all over the world, or to singles resorts where you don't have to worry about a thing and you can be pampered while surrounded by your peers.

The most successful of these is the Club Méditerranée group, with over 80 locations around the world. These informal resorts—from Tahiti to Guadaloupe to North Africa—have developed the reputation of a "swinging" vacation place, but I have been surprised at the large number of married people and parents with children who go to Club Med. My own brother (to whom this book is partially dedicated) and his wife have been to several of them and I hear nothing but glowing reports when they return.

If you're headed overseas on a typical vacation/sight-seeing trip, most singles tours are escorted, just as with any tour group. The advantages are obvious if you are uncomfortable traveling by yourself—companionship, total supervision, guides and airport transportation, and a probable cost advantage (unless we get back to the "singles supplement"). You will, of course, find your way to such groups, and your travel agent or the newspaper ads can help you. It is for the single person who really travels alone that I would like to dedicate the balance of these words of minor wisdom.

TRAVELING ALONE— ALONE

Though on subsequent pages I will specifically address myself to the problems of the woman who travels by herself, there are some general thoughts that really refer to anybody who wants to take off alone or who must travel as a single person. The most important thing, I think, is the *attitude* at the start. What I am saying is that all of us are entitled to proper treatment while traveling, that there is no rule or law or biblical pronouncement that says we must accept improper behavior just because we are alone. I feel, too, that a balance of assertiveness coupled with a sense of humor can do much to make the trip an enjoyable one.

• For any traveler, and especially for the person traveling alone, make sure your hotel reservations are made well in advance, that you specifically request your desires—king-size bed, river view, away from traffic, etc.—and, most important, *that you have a letter from the hotel confirming all of this.* I used to travel to Geneva frequently and I always went there alone and always stayed at the same lovely hotel. Until they began to know me, they haughtily informed me upon arrival that they had no record of the reservation, whereupon I would whip out my letter of confirmation, accept their humble apologies, and be promptly escorted to my room overlooking Lake Lemans.

• Be aware of the fact that hotels overseas do not have the "standard" size American hotel or motel room. When you check in at a Holiday Inn or Marriott Inn in the United States or Canada, you can be certain that the room will be just like the one next door, the one above you, and the one below you. It makes for a feeling of security in knowing exactly what you'll get, but I do find that I wake up in the morning not knowing exactly which city I'm in. Overseas, however, the single rooms are generally quite different from the doubles—usually a converted broom closet that contains a lumpy bed that sags in the middle. After all, you're alone; why on earth would you want elegance? Make sure you specify the kind of room you want when you book. And don't forget that letter of confirmation.

• Single room rates are always comparatively higher than the per-person double occupancy rate. Some hotels around the world charge a fixed fee for the room, regardless of how many share the beds. Just be prepared to spend almost as much for your room as two people who travel together.

• It is generally easier for a single traveler to take advantage of serendipity than it is for a couple. A single ticket to the opera at the last minute, or a seat on a plane that was listed as fully booked, makes leisure time or a change of plans a lot less complicated.

• In restaurants, make sure you make reservations beforehand or, better still, let the concierge make them for you. The hotels generally have more "clout" with restaurants because they will be there to recommend the place long after you've gone. I remember the many times that I have gone into a restaurant on impulse to be greeted by a sea of empty tables, only to be told by the tuxedoed maitre d' that they were all "reserved." My feelings were that they were indeed reserved—but only for more than one person, yet I could never prove it.

• In many cities overseas, the very best restaurant in town is right in the hotel where you are staying. Many of us are too familiar with the usual frozen-glop, microwave fodder that passes as food in most of our domestic motels and franchise restaurants. This is just not so in Europe, so I suggest that you try the restaurant in your hotel if you are on an overseas trip. These are generally geared to the single traveler, and the very fact that you are a guest there will alter the treatment considerably.

• You'll find that by traveling alone you'll meet many more new people than you might if you were traveling in a group or as a couple. Certainly, there are some limitations to this, in the sense of security, and I will cover them more fully in the next section.

• In all of your dealings with hotels, restaurants, taxi drivers, and bellmen, the best thing you can do is to exude an air of confidence and project a feeling that you have done this many times before. Being friendly and open doesn't always work, but you'll be surprised how many times it will get you more attention, better service, and a warm feeling of welcome.

• Don't forget to get the names and addresses of the friends of your friends who might live or work in the city to which you're traveling. Of course, you don't want to "drop in" on them, but a telephone call might lead to a meeting over cocktails or lunch at some lovely restaurant. You might even have your local contacts write before you leave to notify and alert their friends that you will be in their city on a certain date. We have frequently done this, especially for our very young friends who might be leaving on a first trip abroad. It has also resulted in some close and lasting friendships. When your new overseas friends come here to visit, as they no doubt will someday, you can return the hospitality in your own home city.

I might add here that it is very rare for visitors to get invitations to the homes of new acquaintances in some countries. Most entertaining overseas is done outside the home—in local restaurants or cafes. It has nothing to do with you, your personality (we hope), or the fact that you are a visitor. I have traveled and worked in Japan for many years and I have yet to be invited to the home of one of my business acquaintances. I keep telling myself that it has nothing to do with the fact that I am hostile, unfriendly, and gauche. I worked in Italy for two years before I received my first dinner invitation to someone's home. I turned handsprings of joy in the Piazza Navona!

AND FOR THE
WOMAN ALONE

It is getting easier for a lone female to travel in some places, and, as I mentioned earlier, it has not and will never change in others. If you are a woman traveling alone, executive or vacationer, you absolutely must learn as much about your destination as you possibly can. Years ago, when I had my office in Italy, my wife would frequently fly to Rome before me, spend a few days seeing friends or sight-seeing, and then I would join her several days later. The stories she told were horrendous.

Italy is one of those places in the world where any woman alone is fair game for the Lotharios who roam the streets, frequent the restaurants, or are on the lookout for pickups. There are times when it can be entertaining, for the attention and flattery is unusual and many times it's fun and games. My wife tells of one time that a bus came by, crowded with rush-hour passengers. The driver, spotting her walking alongside the bus, leaned forward, and without taking his hands off the wheel, tipped his hat by pushing his head against the windshield. Both of them laughed, the bus went on its way, and it was a harmless flirtation. However at night, the difficulties increased and it was almost impossible to go out to dinner alone without being annoyed or jostled. You must remember that I am an Italophile of the first order—I love Italy and I look forward with bated breath to each return trip. But it is a male-oriented society ("macho" is barely strong enough) and it presents specific problems for the women who travel alone and who want to be left alone.

The same holds true for all of the Arab countries, for Spain, Greece, and Portugal, for all of South America, much of Asia, Turkey, Israel to some extent, and in the hotel and motel lobbies and dining rooms in a great part of the United States and Canada. You absolutely must become familiar with the customs of the country to which you are going. If you can bother to find out that wearing sleeveless dresses in public is frowned upon because of religious customs, then you certainly can take the time to become familiar with the cultural traditions and the roles of women in the society in which you will be a visitor. Any culture that has a deep Latin tradition will probably have an attitude toward women that is less than even-handed. I can name 20 in which the woman is put to death for adultery while the adulterous man is merely exercising his prerogative. So much for progress!

There are some surfacing signs, however, that things may be getting better. The fact is that more and more women are traveling alone, both on business and on vacation. As a result, the travel industry and the tourist offices of various countries have begun to look more closely at this new and potentially rich market. In life, you find that the moment you become part of a "market," people begin to pay more attention to you. This is so if you are a teenager, a natural food aficionado, or just a plain prime-time TV viewer. Thus, women are now a market—and thus, you are now beginning to be heard. The airlines are beginning to pay attention. Domestic and international carriers have all begun to cater to women and to inform them of their travel rights. After all, women executives are now paying passengers who go to every destination in the world. They are also an airline market.

Now booklets are available that cover specific travel recommendations for women—for example, Japan Air Lines' *The Woman's Guide to the Orient.* Seminars are conducted by travel associations and by the airlines themselves, and more travel agents have begun to pay special attention to their female customers. As a matter of fact, nearly 80 percent of all travel agents are women, so there are plenty of sympathetic ears out there. There are also some travel agencies that cater specifically to the woman who travels alone. I recently noticed that there was even a seminar conducted by a New York psychologist on the subject of how to travel alone, and it was specially designed for the woman who has apprehensions about going solo.

Other specific things that may be of assistance if you're a woman setting out alone for the first time:

• Get your travel agent to help by giving you useful and important information. For example, know as much as possible about the hotel to which you're going—whether it's in a safe part of the city, whether transportation is easily available, plus other amenities offered to women. It has been a standing joke in our family that hotel architects and designers have never had to apply make-up in the rooms they've planned. The light is just too dim, the mirror is in the wrong place, or there is no mirror at all.

• In some cities in the world, you may not want to face the dinnertime wolves who roam the streets and restaurants. This is a very real problem, as I indicated with my wife's experiences in Rome. In that case, you might want to have your main meal at lunchtime at that famous restaurant you've always wanted to try, and eat lightly in the evening either at the hotel or at a small restaurant where the management knows you.

A WORD ABOUT SECURITY

In the suggestions that follow, I deal with the matter of security and safety on your trip. But I would like to preface the information with a word of explanation. The more familiar we become with travel, the more open we become to the customs and to the people of the country, the more fun we begin to have, be it woman or man traveling alone. The people we meet and the ideas we exchange are part of what we bring home with us along with our photographs. Indeed, it is part of the reason we go in the first place. The flirtation, the romance, the love affairs, the companionship of people who are strangers at first and grow to be friends are as much a part of the adventure as the first exquisite view of Paris during the "blue hour," that special time at dusk when the city takes on its own color and its own glow.

Conversations, the exchange of ideas, the unforgettable lunch at an outdoor restaurant on the Bosporus—I would be the last person in the world to tell you to pass up any of it. Nevertheless, in the words that follow, I am only suggesting care and warning about naivete. Much of what I say can be taken just as seriously by men as by women. Stay open to your surroundings, keep open to the people you will meet, for what red-blooded American could ever resist an invitation such as the legendary one Charles Boyer murmured, "Come with me to the Casbah." But, back to those suggestions:

• Security is a consideration when you are a woman traveling alone, and thus your agent should recommend a hotel where this is a part of management's concern. The larger hotels are generally quite good about this.

• On the same subject, when you check in, make certain that no one else knows what room has been assigned to you. If the desk clerk calls out your room number too loudly, ask to have it changed.

• Don't open your door to anybody, regardless of what is said on the other side. Use the chain or peephole to confirm that the visitor is who he says he is. If you're in doubt, telephone the front desk or the concierge to ask if anyone was sent up to your room. Many times the interruption is harmless, sometimes the visitor has the wrong room, but you'll want to play it safe. I remember a domestic trip to Atlanta on which our production manager was an attractive blonde. Not 20 seconds after she had closed her door, a male guest, who had been watching through his window as she arrived, knocked on her door. She could not get rid of him, so she telephoned me; I rounded up the three burly males on my crew and we went round to her room. The unwanted visitor left hurriedly and rather sheepishly when he saw us. You, of course, will not have my film crew to call on, so be cautious and be suspicious.

• There is no doubt that women traveling alone are more subject to attention (much of it unwanted) than are men. Certainly, I assume that you are friendly and outgoing, but just be careful of the offers of help with luggage, taxis, or information. There is a tendency for all of us to let our guard down in a foreign country, when our heads are turned by the warmth of the people and the friendliness. But there are dangers that range from confidence games to stolen luggage to actual physical danger. No need to be paranoid—just be careful and circumspect.

I did not forget my dear friends who reminded me to speak of two women traveling together and the treatment they meet along the way. Let me just add that a great many of the tips that I've already given also apply for them, as well as for couples or for families traveling with children. Be affirmative, and be firm. You, too, are a market, just as I am. Don't accept the worst room in the hotel, because you don't have to. No European friend of mine would put up with it. Don't accept the table near the kitchen, and if it takes a small tip to the captain or the maitre d' to move you to the table near the Grand Canal, so be it. It is something that all of us have to put up with at one time or another. Don't let it ruin your trip.

TRAVELING ON A FIXED BUDGET

Before we move on to other things, there is one area of travel that I would like to cover briefly. All of us, business people and vacationers alike, have begun to feel the pinch of rising air fares, hotel prices, the cost of cars, meals, taxis. In business, it is just one of those things that we have to accept and to hope that we can pass it along in the selling price of our products, be they plastics or rental cars.

For many of us, however, the cost of a vacation trip is an economic planning miracle. We want to go, we need the time away, and we make our plans as far in advance as possible. But the prices keep getting in the way. We can travel to Rome for a reasonable amount of money or, by merely changing flight dates, the cost can double all at once. If you are tightly pinched in terms of your travel budget and you look through the ads each Sunday to see the bargains that are offered, the only advice that I can give is: Be careful. Be very, very careful. Ask yourself and your travel agent an awful lot of questions.

Of course, there are bargains to be had, even in these days of inflation and very high travel costs. But many "good deals" hide additional fees, added expenses, penalties for cancellation, and other legalese that makes them less than we bargained for. If we change our minds about the trip, or even if we do arrive as planned, we might find that the "small print" has cost us another $500 that we hadn't expected to spend.

• Read the travel ads and the brochures carefully and ask questions of your travel agent to make sure of what "all-inclusive" means.

• Are rooms double occupancy only? Then what are the surcharges if you want to go alone?

• Watch out for charter flights. There are usually severe penalty cancellation clauses in them. In addition, many charters actually change dates and time of departure at the least provocation. It happened to me several years ago and I had to rebook on a commercial carrier at twice the cost.

• What exactly is included if the tour calls for Modified American Plan or demi-pension? Are you penalized if you decide to take one of your meals outside the hotel? The chances are that you will be. Many ads read: "Includes full continental breakfast." Be aware that this only means you receive orange juice, a roll (possibly a croissant), and coffee. If you're a heavy breakfast eater, add the price of a true breakfast to your costs.

• Even on the air carriers that belong to IATA (International Air Transport Association), as well as on cruise ships, the fare structure changes from day to day, month to month, season to season. By leaving on a weekday you can sometimes save 50 percent of the air fare. Traveling off-season is another way to save money.

• If you must leave on a certain date, ask questions of your agent and the carrier—What are the penalty clauses should you cancel or change? What happens if you make an extra stopover? Many fares are based on direct flights only, and added charges are levied should you decide to make that one short stopover in Paris.

• There is trip cancellation insurance now available through your travel agent or your local insurance broker. Look into it if you are not certain that you can definitely make the flight, or if you want protection against the chance that you might become ill before the trip. The insurance will take care of all cancellation penalties.

• If you're taking a cruise, find out exactly where your cabin will be, if it includes bath or shower, and what extra charges are levied. In other words, is it all-inclusive?

• Of course, liquor and tips are generally not included in most package trips, though occasionally some groups will include tipping that goes with the handling of your luggage at airports and its transfer to the hotel. Again, read the fine print.

For all travelers, there are always hidden costs, and it is good to be prepared for them. There will be entry fees to museums and festivals, tickets to the opera and the theater, that afternoon snack at a cafe. But even if your budget is tight, keep in mind that this trip is one that you've waited for, looked forward to. There is bound to be something that you see that you'll want to buy. There will be some restaurant that you've heard about that you'll want to try. Tuck away some extra money in that secret hideaway of your wallet, just in case you find that something. It will be worth it.

THE
HARRIED
EXECUTIVE

... Dedicated to a Special Breed of Traveler

If you happen to be at an airport, you don't have to be very observant to spot us immediately. We are either carrying attaché cases, or folding clothes bags over our shoulders, or clever overnight bags that will fit snugly under the seat in front of us so we don't have to check our luggage, and all of us have a look that is a combination of experience mixed with the glazed eyes that say: "Do with us what you will."

Some of us hate to travel, some of us love to travel, but *all* of us *must* travel in order to do our jobs properly in this multinational world of ours. And so we make the best of it, even in the worst of times. We try desperately not to travel before, after, or during national holidays, when the vacationer is also on the loose. We try to avoid the airlines if school is just letting out or just getting started, or during intersession. (These days, it seems as if school is always out and we wonder why we are paying tuition for our teenage sons and daughters when we constantly see pictures of them on the beach at Fort Lauderdale.) The spring, summer, and autumn months are the worst, and whether we travel to Europe or anywhere in the United States, every plane seems to be 110 percent filled.

Nevertheless, we have little choice in the matter. We fly when the plane is leaving, close to the hour that we have to go. Indeed, even if we do have an airline of choice, a favorite carrier that still serves champagne, the chançes are that we will never get to fly it, for it either does not go to where we are going, or it does not leave when we must leave. We fly commuter planes, STOL (short takeoff and landing) planes, small jets, and large jets. And if you think that they've crowded the seats closer together in these days of heavy travel (which they have), wait until the next generation of planes arrives! We just completed a film about a new aircraft out on the West Coast, and we found that there is no longer room to walk down the aisle without turning your body sideways. Nevertheless, the airlines and the aircraft manufacturers are already touting the new planes as a step forward. Don't believe a word!

Those who travel for business suffer more weather delays, more fog, more cancellations than any other traveler, for if you fly enough, eventually something that will completely destroy the schedule is bound to happen. On the other hand, we are more travel-wise, more "animal" than any other traveler in the airport, and we can sense a problem immediately with the changing of the departure board.

And through all this, keep one thing in mind—we are also the largest single market for the airline industry, the largest single market for rental cars, long distance credit card calls, hotels and motels, and restaurants. Without us, all of these sellers of services would soon starve.

Without doubt, every one of us could write this chapter in our own way, for each of us has had many of the same experiences, and each of us—man or woman—has developed a hundred personal ways to combat the disease of constant business travel. What follows is what *I* have learned, and, as a result, it reflects the way that I travel when I'm not with my film crews, when I'm off to see a client in some distant city or some Latin American country—my blue denim work shirt (with the epaulets) left at home and my best business suit the "uniform of the day," my black overnight bag slung over my shoulder, and that same glazed airport look in my eye as I wait to check in.

DO YOU REALLY NEED
A TRAVEL AGENT?

As I mentioned earlier, I avoided travel agents for years, merely because I am suspicious and obstinate by nature. Too, each travel agent that I tried managed to fail me in some way. And so I went through the tedium of learning how to read the *Official Airline Guide (OAG)*, wrote countless letters to hotels and waited for just as many confirmations, and generally acted as my own agent. Of course, I have "seen the light," and since I have discovered someone who could put up with my hostile personality, I have turned over to her all of our company's business. There is no doubt that we business people change flights and itineraries more often than any other class of passenger. In our own office, it is not at all unusual for one of our production managers to develop a crew itinerary for six people through seven states over five weeks, only to find, two days before departure, that the film subject is just not available at that time and "Couldn't we change to the week of June 15?" How many business conferences have been shifted, cancelled, rescheduled in your own travel life? Think of all the times you've changed your flights just because you were certain that you could complete your business early the same day and not have to stay overnight in Chicago. It takes a travel agent with the patience of a saint to handle business people, but once you've found that person, don't ever let go!

Nevertheless, it's a good idea to learn how to check and recheck the arrangements made for you. Have a pretty good idea of just what is available *before* you even call the agent, then check the tickets when they arrive at your office. Try, of course, to get confirmed, written, *guaranteed* reservations from your agent before you leave, if time allows. And, most important, try to have an agent who is available to you by long distance telephone during business hours, in case something goes wrong on the trip. Certainly, I have personally jumped up and down on the best hotel desks in the country when my reservation went awry, but I have learned also to call my travel agent at that moment, if the event occurred during business hours, and it frequently has worked out easily. This is particularly good advice when problems arise with the airlines.

If your company has a travel department who books your flights, be particularly careful to double-check the reservation and to read the *OAG* yourself. I have found that many company travel departments have a tendency to book strange connections for their employees, for whatever reasons. Occasionally, I have checked the reservations made by our agent against those of our clients who are to join us at a distant city; noting a discrepancy, I would check the *OAG* and I found time and again that there was an easier and more direct way to get there. Of course, hundreds of letters will now be written to the publisher from irate corporate travel people, but I can only say that I see this occur so often that I must warn you to double-check your itinerary.

THE AIRLINE CLUBS

The airline clubs all have lovely names—Ambassador, Red Carpet, Ionosphere, Senator Lounge, Clipper Club, Horizon, Council Room, Sun King Club—and years ago they were restricted to business people who flew at least a hundred thousand miles a year. No one else could enter, except as a guest. The courts declared this a pure case of discrimination, and they were right. Today, for a small membership fee, anyone can join, and most of you reading this probably already belong to more than one. If you do not, I urge you to look into it.

Of course, you don't want to belong to *all* of them, but you do know which airline you fly the most, which section of the country or the world you visit most often, whether you want a club with only local facilities or one with international ones as a part of their network. In my own case, I belong to only one club, for I fly the airline often and it does, indeed, have both domestic and overseas lounges. For the constantly traveling business person, they can be a boon.

- They provide a sanctuary in times of travel stress—weather delays, long waits between connections, a place for peace and quiet away from the crowded terminal building.

- You can get your seat selected easily and without waiting in line.

- They generally have orange juice, coffee, and sweet rolls available at breakfast time. (I have bowed to my middle-American friends on this; in New York we call sweet rolls "Danish.") Cocktails and soft drinks are also served.

- The telephone booths are comfortable and uncrowded. I cannot understand why all telephones in the United States are now built out in the open, row upon row, one next to the other, with everyone's legs sticking out of the bottom like the corps de ballet. The airport lounges seem to be the only place where you can close a door and hear the other party.

- There are conference rooms available for airport meetings. I remember working for a company once where that seemed to be the only place we'd hold our executive conferences. We'd fly everyone in from San Francisco, New York, Detroit, Atlanta, and Los Angeles and hold the conference at

122

O'Hare Airport in Chicago, then fly them back that same day. I began to feel that our corporation didn't have a home! But it can be convenient.

• Membership is, above all, deductible.

WHAT THE AIRLINES OFFER

We have all realized for years that we pay more than many of our fellow passengers because we are frequently not eligible for the special fares and discounts that are offered and changed daily. How many times have you read the travel pages to find the announcement of a new fare to Europe at half price—but only if you stayed more than 80 days, left on an odd February Wednesday during a leap year, and could return not later than St. Swithin's Day. I am currently going through just such agony in planning a business trip to the south of France, and, in checking the fares, I find with no surprise that I am not eligible for anything except the huge cost of a round trip ticket, with no deductions, no special privileges, no pampering, no sympathy.

If I read these same airline ads, they tell me that I am a "special person," very much in demand (probably because of the fare I pay)—that I will be pampered, petted, made to feel like a king, a lord, a saint, or a Nobel Prize winner; my bags will be stamped, expedited, handled gently, delivered swiftly; and I will arrive at my destination well rested and completely ready to consummate the merger between my small company and General Motors. Of course, once aboard the plane, the bubble will burst and I will no doubt be sitting next to "Steven-put-your-seat-belt-on" and, to make matters worse, Steven will probably be flying free as a part of a fare deal that I cannot use.

Just as I will receive letters of horror from the corporate travel people, I will now get protestations from the airlines telling me that this is just not so any longer, that "things have changed." Well, to an extent they have—or, at the very least, the airlines are trying to change them, for we have complained long enough and loudly enough for them to hear us. But even if the airlines do nothing about it, we still must travel, and they know it.

I remember one airline that promised (for a very short period) that all business people traveling first class would have their luggage stickered as such, and thus they could claim their bags first at the other end. I tried the airline, based on this promise and on the fact that they were leaving when I had to go. The results were predictable. In Los Angeles, the bags arrived last—not next-to-last but *last,* on a plane that had carried over 350 passengers! There are times—too many of them, perhaps—when the airlines cannot deliver what they promise and they know it. This particular experiment lasted about one month and I have not heard the airline mention it since.

But there are other things that the airlines offer business people, and some of them do work, and some of them are worth taking advantage of on your longer trips. They change from month to month, but a quick check of the airline of your choice will tell you just what is in vogue at that moment. Currently, there are many things being attempted:

First Class. Of course, the surcharge is worth looking into, either to force you back into economy class or to justify it to yourself by planning to get your work done in relative ease, comfort, and peace and quiet. Many corporations have cut back on first-class travel, and with good reason. But I have found that on certain trips the surcharge is well worth the trade-off of work or reading that I can do.

Sleeper Seats. These also carry a large surcharge. Some airlines have even expanded them into small berths, much like the sleeperettes of train travel. Again, if you are going overseas and you have an important meeting coming up when you arrive (and more on that later), it might be worth your while, if the company permits, to book one of these sleepers. The first time I ever tried a sleeper seat was on a long flight from New York to Rio de Janeiro, and the difference was astounding. Another time, while traveling to India, the flight attendants kept waking me up to feed, pamper, and talk to me, so the sleeper might just as well have been a regular seat.

Business Peoples' Sections. This is a fairly new innovation and it's called by various names—Business Class, the Tachibana Cabin, Clipper Class. It's where the full-fare passenger is separated from the others in a separate cabin, usually in the middle of the plane right behind first class and in front of the last coach cabin. The airlines promise that, if at all possible, a seat will be left empty between passengers to allow for more room to work or to relax, but I have found that in these days of crowded aircraft, almost every seat is occupied on almost every flight. The most important benefit for the full-fare business passenger, however, is that it keeps the children away while you're working.

There are other things that the airlines have attempted to do in order to ease the burden of the business traveler:

- Some offer a separate check-in in addition to the separate section of the plane.

- Some give the same overseas baggage allowance as that of the first-class passengers (66 pounds).

- Free headsets for the movie, free cocktails, and early service at meal-time may be provided.

- Various airlines will make your car rental and hotel service reservations. As I've already mentioned, I am suspicious of anyone but my travel agent (double-checked by me) in making hotel or car rental accommodations.

- Some airlines will make arrangements for printing your business cards in a foreign language. Just allow enough time, for it may take several weeks.

- Some airline offices overseas can act as your local mail pickup and delivery center. This can help tremendously if you are not going to be in one spot for any length of time. Hotels are notorious for not delivering mail that has been addressed to you and has arrived before you. (And this is the place that angry hotel managers will write to my publisher, but wait until they see Chapter 22!)

- Some flights going overseas now have radio-telephones aboard. For those of you who, like me, cannot keep away from the infernal machine, this is a boon. In fact, I am on the telephone so often that one of my clients has begun to call me "Mel Bell."

- Many overseas carriers are now offering special lounges and offices where you can go for information, desk space, secretarial help, typewriters, calculators, and photocopying machines. The latter have been of tremendous help to me, since I have been constantly frustrated in trying to make copies of my important documents while traveling overseas.

Before you leave, it's also a good idea to check the airlines to see if they have published anything that might be of use to you on your business trip. Of course, the best contact and source of information overseas is your own business associate in your company—someone who lives at the destination and who, hopefully, speaks the language. On the latter point, I have found,

125

unfortunately, too many Americans who have lived overseas for 10 to 20 years and who barely speak the language of the country. What makes matters worse is that they're proud of it!

There are the standard travel books, and my shelf is filled with them, but the literature I am speaking of is the "specialty" booklet that deals with a specific subject and is addressed to the business man or woman. One of the best overall guides that I've used is the hardcover book *Pan Am's World Guide* (McGraw-Hill, New York, 1976, $7.95). The reason I like it is that it gives its information succinctly and it covers areas such as electric current, tipping, restaurants, currency, and hotels. There are, of course, others—some of them free and some available at nominal cost from the airline. SAS, for example, provides a free booklet called *Business Travelers' Guide to Scandinavia.* Japan Air Lines, whose books carry a small charge, produces *Businessman's After Hours Guide to Japan, Executive Guide to the Orient,* and *Business in Japan.* These are but a few examples. I suggest that you write to the airlines and ask for their lists of publications devoted to business travel, as well as to the special services they offer.

A few years ago our own company was involved in an interesting project geared to the expanding business relations between Japanese and American companies. We produced a motion picture in conjunction with BCIU (Business Council for International Understanding) called *Doing Business in Japan.* With the cultural differences between the two countries so vast, we felt that there was a deep need for such a film, for Americans and Japanese alike were finding it almost impossible to bridge the gaps that appeared when they tried to do business together. A great many corporations now use the film as an orientation tool for executives who are about to take their first trip, or to be transferred, to Japan. (For information on rental fees, you can write to our office: Vision Associates, 665 Fifth Avenue, New York, NY 10022.)

AN EXECUTIVE EMERGENCY TRAVEL KIT

And finally, if I may, I'd like to list just a few of the tips that I've picked up over my years of travel. Some may be familiar and others may make you sit up in wonder and ask why you didn't think of them before. I am still collecting them on all my trips and in my conversations with business people—and possibly, by the fifth edition of *Easy Going,* some of your vital tips will be included and the list will have grown to astronomical proportions.

• On short trips, most of us try not to take luggage that has to be checked through, especially when there is a connection involved. With the cleverly designed bags today and the folding, hanging, soft clothing bag, I can frequently travel for two to three days without taking a large piece of luggage. And it sure helps when you have a tight connection and the wait for luggage seems to take as long as the trip.

• In addition to your regular needs, and considering that everyone has his or her own "emergency" kit, you might look at this list to see if anything on it might also help you:

Folding raincoat.

Sewing kit.

Slippers.

Business cards.

Letterhead stationery and envelopes.

Carbon paper (in case you can't find a photocopy machine).

Scotch tape.

Paper clips.

Official Airline Guide (or photocopied pages from a complete edition).

OAG Pocket Planner (a handy publication listing hotels and restaurants).

• If you travel internationally, keep your immunizations up to date, even if you have not taken an overseas trip for some time. The last thing you want is to discover two days before your trip that you need a yellow fever shot, plus typhoid and tetanus boosters!

• Know your travel options before you leave. In other words, in addition to carrying the pocket *OAG,* study the alternatives in case of delay or cancellation when you get to the airport. It will save time and possibly get you the last seat on the next flight should you have to make the last-minute change.

• As I mentioned before, check your tickets when they arrive from your agent or your corporate travel office. I remember failing to do just that about ten years ago when I went on vacation to Spain and discovered to my horror (while standing in a plaza in Seville) that my agent (no longer my agent) had pulled the wrong coupon out of my ticket book and I was left without transportation back to the United States. I spent five days going back and forth to the airline office until it was settled. It took four cables, three overseas calls, and 27 stumbling arguments in Spanish before they gave me the replacement ticket. I now read my ticket stubs more carefully, you can be sure.

• Don't forget a list of home telephone numbers, and those of your business associates and friends at your final destination as well as all along the route. You never know when you'll need them—and it may be at a time when your office is closed.

• Try to reconfirm your meetings before you leave, or as soon as you arrive. I don't know how many times I've walked into an office in Latin America to be greeted with, "Oh, is today the day?" This has happened even after I had reconfirmed by cable.

• I cover hotel guarantees in Chapter 22, but try to have all confirmations in writing if you can. It helps, if you arrive at the desk and they can't "remember" your reservation.

• Check out the need for car rental carefully. Sometimes it just doesn't pay to rent a car, and taxis are easier and more convenient. Try to know the airport—is it difficult to get a car? (Try Miami in season!) I seldom rent one in Washington, D.C., unless I'm going into the suburbs of Virginia or Maryland. It takes forever to get a car and taxis are cheaper. Of course, in Los Angeles you must have a car in order to get around, and in Detroit the taxi fares and distances will bankrupt your company; parking in New York is almost impossible, and Chicago is a tossup.

• Overseas car rental will be determined by many factors: Do they drive on the left or right? Can you read the signs? In Japan, all signs are in the Japanese language only. Check with your travel agent or the local contact in the city to which you're going before you make up your mind. I drive in England, Yugoslavia, and most of Africa, but I would not rent a car without a driver in India or Japan.

• If you're going overseas, try to travel during daylight hours, as suggested in an earlier chapter. I notice in the newspapers that more and more political figures are now arriving in the United States on Saturday or early Sunday, allowing them time to adjust to jet lag before attending their Monday meetings. The business person could well learn from them. If you can't travel during the day, try to take a daylight flight to a major point, such as London, and then make the early-morning connection to the continent. If the trip is much longer, try not to have a business meeting on arrival, if you can help it. Get plenty of rest before you meet with your associates. You may wake up one morning to find that you've sold your company without knowing it.

• A word about the "Red Eye Specials" of the world. These are the overnight flights that (for example) leave Los Angeles at 10:45 P.M. and arrive in New York at about 6:00 A.M. eastern standard time. I avoid them if I can. They're debilitating, tiring, and unnecessary. It's time that we business people traveled on business hours.

• And a new piece of airline propaganda caught my eye recently—an abomination that suggests that we travel *overseas* on a two-day, round-trip schedule! My jaw hung open as I read that they are now suggesting we take the morning flight to London, get a good night's sleep, have our meeting the next day, and then return *that evening* to New York. And they call it "a businessman's dream," which leads me to believe that *businesswomen* are too smart to attempt the trip. Rubbish! No wonder so many executives expire at an early age.

• Speaking (however derogatorily) of the airlines, it is a good idea to check in early and to get your seat assignment, and then to board the aircraft as early as possible. You have discovered, as have I, that computers are not infallible; in the past two years, I have been the victim of double-booking of seats no less than six times. Each time, though, I was the first one in the seat of a completely sold-out flight, and each time it was the other person who had to work it out with the agent.

• I watch the departure information at the airport rather carefully and there is one "red flag" that I shudder to see. If your flight suddenly has a departure time changed and the symbol reads "See Agent," it is generally an indication that the flight has been cancelled or delayed for a long period of time. "Get thee to another airline" or make some kind of arrangement for booking another flight. Don't delay, for generally there are too few seats on the next flight anyway.

• Incidentally, there is one Civil Aeronautics Board rule that you should be familiar with. When a flight is delayed and the time is then changed to a later departure, the flight *cannot* leave any earlier than the new posted time. As a result, the airlines will generally post a new "optimistic" time because of a mechanical failure or a late arrival, hoping that they can get you out by then. That is one of the reasons that the delays usually take much longer than the new time of departure would indicate. If they should post a new time that was two hours later and the mechanical problem was fixed in an hour, they still could not leave until the posted time.

• Call the airline before you leave town for the flight. This is important if the weather is especially bad. On international travel, remember that all airlines still carry the 72-hour reconfirmation rule. You must reconfirm or your reservation will be automatically cancelled. And do it early! I remember arriving in Lisbon on a trip from Yugoslavia, and the airline that brought me into Portugal was the one I was to take back to the United States several days later. Arriving at my hotel, I decided to reconfirm my flight home. The airline had automatically cancelled my reservation because they had no record that I was even on their flight that had just arrived an hour before from Yugoslavia; obviously, I didn't exist. Of course, they apologized and blamed it on—guess what—the computer.

• Do your expense report every day, or every two days. I'm sure you find, as I do, that if you let it go too long, you can't remember whether you spent the money for dinner, for a taxi, or for a bullfight. Just makes notes if it's too much trouble to make out the entire report. How many business people have you seen on the return flights juggling little slips of paper and trying to figure out whether the rate of exchange was 24 rupees to one dollar or, come to think of it, was it 24 French francs?

There is one other thing that every business person should pack as a part of the trip—and it is also good advice for any traveler. Take along your sense of humor. I remember running into an old friend of mine three separate times in one week, each time at an airport. He, too, is in the film business and he travels just about the same number of miles as I do each year. We met by accident at John F. Kennedy Airport in New York, then ran into each other in the corridors of O'Hare in Chicago, and then two days later at a check-in counter in Los Angeles. We laughed and he shook his head, "I guess we're all migrant workers, aren't we?" And so we are.

12

BE IT EVER SO HUMBLE—THERE'S NO NEED TO STAY HOME

Travel with Diabetes, Accommodation for the Blind Traveler, the Deaf Traveler— and the Traveler on Wheels

When I began to research this chapter, I was thoroughly convinced that it would be the most difficult one for which to get complete information and the most complex for which to acquire printed materials, articles from newspapers, and assistance from the medical profession and the travel industry. I suppose my mind was placed somewhere around 20 years back, when this would have been true.

To my delighted surprise, each inquiry led to still another source of information, and my office began to look as though the public library had been cleaned out and the material stacked near my typewriter. As I write, the floor and sofa are piled high with books, pamphlets, articles, personal letters, suggestions, government documents, literature from the airlines, bus lines, cruise lines, railroads, and travel agents. Travel for the handicapped? I have brochures that offer trips to Hawaii, Mexico, Europe, Africa, and Alaska. It is my honest belief, as the mail continues to pour in, that there is more literature and more advice available for the traveler with a physical disability than for any other subject area covered in this book!

SOME VERY
SPECIAL PEOPLE

It was, of course, not always so, and I learned this rather quickly when I began to read the material that was sent to me. It is only in the past few years that the travel industry and government tourist organizations have begun to realize that people with physical handicaps need not stay at home—indeed, that they do not *want* to stay at home. Finally, the people who have the power to move things have begun to do something about it, and as a result, the world has become more accessible. In many instances, the law has been amended to provide access for the handicapped.

In an article written for the *ICTA Journal* (Institute of Certified Travel Agents), Winter 1979, Alathena Miller tells of her travels in a wheelchair for over 30 years—around the world four times, twice alone, her trip to Machu Picchu (a difficult one for any traveler), to the top of the Acropolis, and down the 99 steps of the Catacombs in Alexandria, Egypt. My own editor through three of my books, Charles Gerras, has never let his wheelchair become a barrier to his travel plans and, in fact, many of the tips in the last part of this chapter are his very good advice, culled from his own personal experiences.

The subject is, to be sure, a vast one. And it is still complex; I do not mean to make it sound easy. The preplanning necessary for the trip is sometimes quite involved. The rules and regulations vary from airline to airline, from country to country. But the important thing is that information and help is now available as never before. The experts have written their own books, the doctors have taken a hand in getting their patients out on vacations that were once just dreams, and the very same materials that now lie storm-strewn over my office floor are also available to you. If you are an experienced traveler in spite of your physical disability, then there is probably little that I can add. If you have never traveled much, for whatever reason, I think I can be of help.

What I try to do in the pages that follow is to pick out the important tips for those of you who want to travel but are anxious about making the next move. And then, throughout the chapter and at the very end, I list sources for further information, a way to find the people and the support you may need to set off on a journey to almost anywhere, given some limitations. You might also note that, because of this growing market, more and more travel agents are beginning to provide special tours and special assistance to the physically handicapped traveler, and I have added a listing of some of the best in the field.

IF YOU ARE UNDER THE DOCTOR'S CARE

If your physical disability is such that you have been under a doctor's care, you certainly will want a consultation before you even begin to make your plans. If, for example, you are using medication, make certain you have enough of it with you to last the entire trip. In addition, have your doctor give you a prescription that can be filled anywhere along the way—and know the *generic* name of the drug you are taking. Keep in mind that many of the pharmaceuticals in this country are dispensed by trade name, depending upon the manufacturer. Not only are you paying too much for them as a result, but you probably won't be able to get them overseas. And if you are taking medications with you, make sure you carry them right on your person rather than packing them in your luggage. It's also a good idea to carry a copy of the prescription or a note from your doctor along with you, since many countries are terribly suspicious of little bottles filled with white powders.

Organizations such as IAMAT (International Association for Medical Assistance to Travelers) and Medic Alert (see Chapter 20) also have warning tags printed for emergencies that might possibly occur while you are on your trip.

Check the weather and the altitude at your final destination and at all stops along the way. People with diabetes and arthritis, for example, are particularly susceptible to cold weather, and frostbite can be a dangerous problem if it occurs. Though high altitudes can affect any traveler, people who have been under treatment for cardiovascular conditions should be particularly careful. Under normal conditions, any person who can climb a flight of stairs or walk a short distance without undue adverse symptoms can usually fly on today's commercial jets. On the other hand, since cabin pressures are set between 5,000 and 7,000 feet, patients just recovering from coronaries are

Opposite, traveler's clinical record provided by International Association for Medical Assistance to Travelers (IAMAT)

134

*If your patient is taking
Anticoagulant drugs for
a Cardio-Vascular condition
please have him sign the card below:*

ALERT!

name (print): _____

signature _____

I am taking anticoagulant drugs

If I am involved in an accident or found unconscious,
take me to the hospital immediately.

I am undergoing treatment with_____
_____ name brand of anticoagulant and dosage

Prothrombin Time Test and Anticoagulant Dosage Record

Date	Prot. time patient	Prot. time control	Hematuria*	Dosage until next blood test	Physician's Signature

*Record: O (Absent) — G (Gross) — M (Microscopic). The numerals
following M indicate the number of red cells present in the microscopic
field.

135

generally advised to wait at least three to four months before embarking on a journey by plane. Cities such as Denver, Mexico City, Bogota, Cuzco, or Quito may well be on your doctor's avoidance list if you have been suffering from a heart condition. Once again, the good advice is to check with your family physician long before you make your plans.

Whatever the physical problem, then, be it diabetes or heart condition, arthritis, or even a simple allergy, the important thing is that you do your homework before you go. If there are special problems of access or special needs, the advice goes doubly for hotels, transportation, local cars and buses, sight-seeing, and guided tours. Everything must be checked out well in advance.

TRAVELING WITH DIABETES

There is a superb little pamphlet available for diabetic patients who want to travel, and what follows is taken directly from it (with permission, of course). It's called *Vacationing with Diabetes, Not from Diabetes* and it was written by Dr. Samuel Mirsky, past chairman of the New York Diabetes Association and now on the attending staff of Mount Sinai, Lenox Hill, and Doctors Hospitals in New York. It is available through your local diabetes association, or by writing directly to E. R. Squibb & Sons, P.O. Box 4000, Lawrenceville-Princeton Road, Princeton, NJ 08540. I strongly suggest that you send for it if you are planning your vacation. Dr. Mirsky recommends that:

• You have an identification card, bracelet, or necklace stating that you are under treatment for diabetes and are taking insulin.

• You get your medical checkup and vaccines before you leave.

• You take emergency medication with you: glucagon, antidiarrheal medication, antiemetic for nausea prevention, suntan lotion with para-aminobenzoic acid.

• You take emergency carbohydrates on the trip, such as Life Savers, sugar cubes, and liquid glucose.

• You not forget urine and blood testing devices.

- You have enough of your own oral drug or insulin to last the trip.

- You take with you some regular insulin for an emergency even if you are taking long-acting medicine.

- You get a note from your doctor describing your diabetic condition and explaining the medicines and the needles you are carrying.

In addition, Dr. Mirsky feels, and I agree, that it's a good idea to learn enough emergency terms in the language of the country to which you're going so that you're able to explain your condition, the medication you are taking, and any other allergies you may have. He also lists the foreign equivalents for the oral drugs sold in the United States, some tips on crossing time zones (especially since you will be taking medication on a regular basis), information about diet, emergencies, and a warning about staying away from native "cures" for diabetes. It is a marvelous booklet.

In an earlier chapter, I mentioned an item that I always take with me on my trips—a small, throwaway flashlight (even though I must say again that I am disturbed by any society that wastes something by throwing it away). But the flashlight is quite small, easy to carry in a pocket or purse, and it's most valuable for those late night calls to the dark bathroom. Since it is potentially harmful for diabetics to bruise themselves—and a sleepy trip in the dark might well result in an injury—you might want to pack one in your luggage or in your hand-carried bag.

There is also a nationwide club for diabetic travelers that might be of help to you if you're setting off on a trip. It's the DTS Club (Diabetes Travel Service, Inc.), located at 349 East Fifty-second Street, New York, NY 10022. They have a small membership fee of $15 per year ($25 for two years), and they offer travel tips, guidance about food, and special identification cards. They also can help to locate group tours, books, and merchandise such as special insulin travel kits at discount prices.

THE
BLIND TRAVELER

In Chapter 9, I discussed travel with pets, and I noted that there are some countries such as Australia and Great Britain that will not allow dogs or cats into the country without a long period of quarantine. Unfortunately, this law also applies to guide dogs and they will make no exceptions at all. As a result, it's a good idea to check the rules of the country thoroughly before making any plans for travel. Even if your guide dog should be admitted, make certain that you carry a slip or certificate stating that the animal has been inoculated against rabies and is in general good health.

When you travel with a guide dog, most carriers will allow you to take the animal right on board with you, where it can lie on the floor between your feet during the trip. However, various airlines have different rules about this, and many times the decision will depend upon how long the trip is going to be. Make certain that you or your travel agent notify the airline when your reservation is made. Buses and trains present no problem.

When I discussed this with Pat McKee of the Lighthouse for the Blind, she strongly suggested that you take your vacation trips with a companion, whether you use a guide dog or travel with a cane. If you're not with a group that is specially geared to your needs, she says: ". . . don't expect to find a guardian angel on your trip. Certainly, someone will cross the street with you and help you occasionally, but no stranger will sacrifice his good time on a trip to cater to your needs. Take a friend or a relative along."

Incidentally, the major bus lines such as Greyhound, Trailways, and Continental all provide free transportation for the companion of a handicapped person, provided that you can prove the need for that person. However, those traveling with a guide dog *and* a sighted companion, or two blind persons traveling together, are not eligible. The railroads have also made arrangements for companions of handicapped people, usually at a reduced fare. You will probably have to present written proof of your need; the American Foundation for the Blind will provide a permanent card along with a list of bus lines and railroads that grant the concessions. There is a small fee: $2.50 for the identification card and $1.25 for a coupon book that some carriers require for travel in exchange for tickets. You will also have to submit three recent 1¼" x 1½", full-face, close-up photographs of yourself, plus a certification—from an ophthamologist, a physician, an optometrist, or an executive of an agency for the blind—that your vision status makes you eligible. For further information, you can write to: Travel Concession, American Foundation for the Blind, 15 West Sixteenth Street, New York, NY 10011. Regional offices of the foundation in Chicago, Atlanta, Denver, and San Francisco will also process your request.

If you're off on a first trip to Europe or across the country, and you've decided to go with a group tour, make sure the travel agency has had experience in this area. The very good ones have made it a point to hire guides who have a talent for word pictures of the places they visit. Some tour leaders purchase models of the landmarks they visit, such as the Empire State

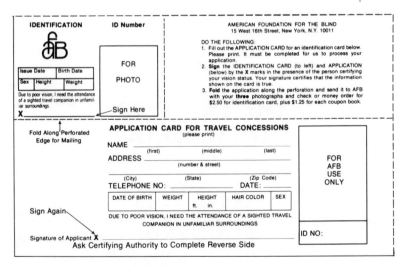

CERTIFICATION OF POOR VISION

To be completed by an ophthalmologist, physician, optometrist, an executive of an agency for the blind, or other competent authority.

Indicate for each eye, after best correction:
a) degree of visual acuity in SNELLEN measurements
b) field of vision
c) whether the individual has light perception

Fold Along Perforated Edge for Mailing

AMERICAN FOUNDATION FOR THE BLIND, INC.
15 West 16th Street, New York, N.Y. 10011
212-620-2177 Travel Concession Program

Use of this Card to Obtain Travel Concession

This card identifies the holder as having been certified by an ophthalmologist, physician, optometrist, executive of an agency for the blind or other competent authority as having limited vision. Documentation is on file at the American Foundation for the Blind. Under the amendments of the Interstate Commerce Act of 1927, a person who is disabled or whose vision is so limited as to need the attendance of a sighted companion when traveling in unfamiliar surroundings may be granted reduced fares on interstate carriers. A list of these carriers is on record at AFB.

Loyal E. Apple, Executive Director

PLEASE RETURN TO THE HOLDER IF FOUND

RIGHT EYE
a) visual acuity: _____
b) visual field: _____
c) light perception: ___ Yes ___ No

LEFT EYE
a) visual acuity: _____
b) visual field: _____
c) light perception: ___ Yes ___ No

Signed _____   Title _____   Date _____

Name of Agency _____   Address _____

FOR AFB USE ONLY

Proof of blindness card

IDENTIFICATION   **ID Number**

FOR PHOTO

Sign Here

Issue Date | Birth Date
Sex | Height | Weight

Due to poor vision, I need the attendance of a sighted travel companion in unfamiliar surroundings.

X

Fold Along Perforated Edge for Mailing

AMERICAN FOUNDATION FOR THE BLIND
15 West 16th Street, New York, N.Y. 10011

DO THE FOLLOWING:
1. Fill out the APPLICATION CARD for an identification card below. Please print. It must be completed for us to process your application.
2. **Sign** the IDENTIFICATION CARD (to left) and APPLICATION (below) by the X marks in the presence of the person certifying your vision status. Your signature certifies that the information shown on the card is true.
3. **Fold** the application along the perforation and send it to AFB with your **three** photographs and check or money order for $2.50 for identification card, plus $1.25 for each coupon book.

APPLICATION CARD FOR TRAVEL CONCESSIONS
(please print)

NAME _____
(first)   (middle)   (last)

ADDRESS _____
(number & street)

(City)   (State)   (Zip Code)

TELEPHONE NO: _____   DATE: _____

DATE OF BIRTH | WEIGHT | HEIGHT ft. in. | HAIR COLOR | SEX

Sign Again

DUE TO POOR VISION, I NEED THE ATTENDANCE OF A SIGHTED TRAVEL COMPANION IN UNFAMILIAR SURROUNDINGS

Signature of Applicant X _____

Ask Certifying Authority to Complete Reverse Side

FOR AFB USE ONLY

ID NO:

Card for blind travel discount

Building or the Eiffel Tower, and the blind travelers can feel the shape with their fingers as the structure is being described.

AND FOR THE DEAF TRAVELER

Since the deaf traveler does not have an obvious handicap so far as the rest of the world is concerned, help is just not as readily available as it might be for the person who is blind or one who is confined to a wheelchair.

Again, it is wise to notify the airline on which you're traveling, beginning with your check-in at the ticket counter and again aboard the plane. I have found that many messages given to agents never get to the flight crew in the rush to depart on time (which no one seems to do anymore anyhow). Flight attendants have been trained to give written emergency instructions to flyers who are deaf, and to notify them of any announcements that are made during the flight. The airports now have amplified telephones available for the hard of hearing, but flight announcements, weather delays, cancellations are generally given over the airport loudspeakers and can be missed by someone who is deaf. While you're waiting for your plane, keep an eye on the monitor screens that are usually posted around the airport terminal and near the lounges. If there is a delay, it will generally be posted on that monitor.

The same rules and regulations that are in effect for guide dogs for the blind are now beginning to be accepted for hearing ear dogs. With proper identification and validation of the need for the dog, they are generally allowed to sit right with the passenger on the bus, the train, and on most airlines.

THE TRAVELER ON WHEELS

I mentioned earlier that there is a vast amount of literature available for the handicapped traveler, and I have listed some of the better pamphlets and books at the end of this chapter. It would be a simple matter for me to merely research my treasure trove of materials and excerpt the tips from what already exists. My hope, though, has been to keep this book as personal as possible, and if the experiences have been mine, I have recounted them (and in the recounting I have no doubt embellished them). If the experiences have been those of my friends and coworkers, I have gladly accepted their stories and their tips for inclusion in the book. For each of us can learn from the other, and my own travel "savvy" continues to grow as I listen.

In this case, my own editor, Charles Gerras, is an experienced wheelchair traveler and has been flying around the world for years. Through telephone conversations, personal discussions, and many hilarious exchanges of travel tales, I've compiled a list of tips that Charlie has given to me over these past few months. In addition, I've also included a personal log of his recent trip aboard the QE-2.

Certainly, there are many details to consider, depending upon where you're going and how you're going to get there. But, in perusing his list and then reading the materials that lie piled before me, I realized that Charlie has managed to cull the most important points and put them into a concise sequence. After all, he is a superb editor, so that is the least that I can expect of him!

Primarily, when you're traveling in a wheelchair, you absolutely must take the initiative. You just cannot depend upon people to realize the problems you encounter in doing things that are ordinary for everyone else. In planning your trip, think it through thoroughly. Travel agents who have not had experience with booking physically disabled people generally cannot be depended upon to anticipate your needs. That, and the fact that most travel literature for the handicapped has been written by able-bodied people, puts the burden of making the trip a success in your lap. Of course, if you are a part of a group that is being run by experienced travel experts, and all access, accommodations, transportation, and sight-seeing will be taken care of by them, you can relax somewhat. But if you are traveling with a companion and are setting off on your own, read carefully:

AIRPLANES

Some carriers, depending upon the type of aircraft being used, will limit the number of passengers who are physically handicapped. This means that you should make your flight reservations as far in advance as possible, and let the airline know your needs. Incidentally, the airlines also have rules as to who may or may not travel without a companion, so this is another thing worth checking in advance.

• If possible, get the wide-bodied 747 jet. At the entry door of this plane there are three seats that are perfectly situated for handicapped travelers. You wheel through the door and right to the seat—no need to transfer to a boarding chair to get down the aisle. (No airliner aisle is wide enough to accommodate a full-size wheelchair, so you will have to use the high-back, narrow boarding chairs to get to your seat.)

Airlines require that the wheelchair be stowed during flight, so don't plan to use it as your seat. When you are booked on flights with the smaller aircraft, such as the DC-9, and where there is no boarding jetway to the plane, you will have to use the boarding chair to get onto the plane via the portable stairway. Don't let that keep you from going—the airline personnel are courteous and ever ready to help. If at all possible, however, book your originating flights and your connecting flights through major gateways, since the service available for access is much greater.

- If the wheelchair can be put aboard with you, so much the better. However, if it must be stowed, keep in mind that you will have to get to the baggage carousel once you leave the plane. Without your wheelchair you can't get there to pick up your wheelchair! They might not make that connection—you must! Make sure the wheelchair will be accessible to you when the plane reaches the ramp. Most airlines will make sure that the wheelchair is plucked out of the regular baggage group or stowed up front in the cabin so it can be given to you at the plane after all the other passengers have disembarked. This is particularly vital to you if your wheelchair is specially designed for you. You may have to insist that one of the all-purpose airline terminal wheelchairs simply will not do.

Airlines also have different rules and regulations concerning the boarding of batteries, whether wet or dry. Also make sure that you check this out if your wheelchair is battery-powered.

- Get to the airport well ahead of departure time, so that all your needs can be met. Normally, airlines recommend about an hour between your arrival time at the airport and departure of the plane (less on domestic flights). However, don't forget to figure traffic to the airport, rush hour crush, special needs, access to the terminal and preboarding at the gate. I suggest arrival at least an hour and a half to two hours before plane time.

There is a booklet published by the U.S. Department of Transportation that may be of help to you at the airport. It's called *Access Travel: Airports,* and it's free. Write to: Architectural and Transportation Barriers Compliance Board, 330 "C" Street, S.W., Washington, DC 20201. If you'd like multiple copies of the book for your club or group, write to: Office of Public Affairs, APA-400, Federal Aviation Administration, 800 Independence Avenue, S.W., Washington, DC 20591.

• If you cannot utilize the toilets aboard the aircraft for physical reasons, make sure you do not take any fluids for 12 hours before the flight, if possible.

• If you can walk, make sure the seat assignment is near one of the lavatories, so that you don't have to make your way down the long aisle. On today's 747s, it can be quite a hike.

BUS AND TRAIN TRAVEL

With the implementation of special programs for the handicapped, travel aboard buses and trains has gotten somewhat easier for those who use a wheelchair. The major bus lines have instituted programs that range from free fares for traveling companions to new terminal facilities that include larger doorways, restrooms, telephones, water fountains, food service areas, handrails, and ramps that are designed for the physically disabled. Some of the carriers, such as Greyhound, are designing their new buses with "kneeling steps" for easier access. Before you set off, check Greyhound, Trailways, and Continental,

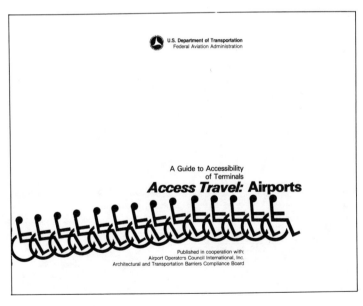

Travel access manual for airports

Interior spread from *Access Travel: Airports*

	ABERDEEN SCOTLAND	AGANA GUAM	ALBANY GA	ALBUQUERQUE NM	ALGER ALGERIA
PARKING					
PARKING SPACES RESERVED FOR HANDICAPPED	•	•	S	•	
DIRECTIONAL SIGNING TO RESERVED SPACES		•	S	•	
SPACES LEVEL AND AT LEAST 12 FEET WIDE	•	•	S	•	
SPACES WITHIN 200 FEET OF TERMINAL ENTRANCE	•	•	S	•	
SPACES PROTECTED FROM WEATHER				•	
PARKING METERS AND TICKETS ACCESSIBLE TO DRIVER	•	NA	•	•	•
LEVEL OR RAMPED PATH FROM PARKING TO ENTRANCE	•	•	•	•	•
EXTERIOR CIRCULATION					
VEHICULAR AND PASSENGER TRAFFIC SEPARATED	•	•	•	•	
ALL WALKWAYS AT LEAST 5 FEET WIDE	NA	•	•	•	S
STAIRS AND RAMPS AT ALL CHANGES OF LEVEL	NA	NA	•		•
HANDRAILS ON ALL RAMPS AND STAIRS	•	NA	NA		•
CURB CUTS AT ALL PEDESTRIAN CROSSINGS	•	•	•	•	
ALL RAMPS AT LEAST 5 FEET WIDE	•	NA	•		NA
ALL RAMP SLOPES 8.3% OR LESS	NA	NA	•	•	NA
ALL RAMPS INDICATED BY ACCESSIBILITY SYMBOL	•	NA			NA
ALL RAMPS PROTECTED FROM SNOW AND ICE		NA	NA	NA	NA
ALL RAMP SURFACES NON-SLIP	•	•	•	•	NA
RAMPS OVER 30 FEET LONG HAVE LEVEL REST LANDINGS	NA	NA	NA	NA	NA
RAMPS HAVE LEVEL LANDINGS AT TURNS	NA	NA	•	•	NA
RAMPS HAVE HANDRAILS ON BOTH SIDES	NA	NA	NA		NA
ARRIVAL AND DEPARTURE					
LEVEL VEHICLE LOADING/UNLOADING AREAS CLOSE TO BLDG ENTRANCES	•	NA	•	•	•
LOADING/UNLOADING AREAS PROTECTED FROM WEATHER	NA			•	
INTERIOR CIRCULATION					
BUILDING ENTRANCES AND EXITS LEVEL WITH AUTOMATIC DOOR	•	•		•	
PUBLIC AREAS IN BUILDING ACCESSIBLE BY LEVEL/RAMPED ROUTE	•	•	•	•	S
PUBLIC CORRIDORS AT LEAST 5 FEET WIDE AND OBSTRUCTION FREE	•	•	•	•	•
ELEVATORS					
PUBLIC ELEVATORS ACCESSIBLE ON LEVEL PATH	•	NA	NA	•	•
PUBLIC ELEVATORS TO ALL FLOORS, INCLUDING GARAGE	NA	NA	NA	NA	
ELEVATORS AT LEAST 5 BY 5 FEET INSIDE MEASUREMENT	NA	NA	NA	•	
ELEVATOR DOOR OPENING AT LEAST 3 FEET	•	NA	NA	•	•
ELEVATOR DOORS HAVE AUTOMATIC SAFETY REOPENING DEVICE	•	NA	NA	•	•
ELEVATOR CONTROLS NO MORE THAN 4 FEET ABOVE FLOOR	•	NA	NA		•
ELEVATOR CONTROLS HAVE RAISED LETTERING		NA	NA	•	•
STAIRS					
RAMP OR ELEVATOR AVAILABLE AS ALTERNATE TO STAIRS OR ESCALATORS	NA	NA	NA	•	S
STAIRWAYS FREE OF PROJECTING NOSES	NA	NA	NA	•	S
STAIRWAY RISER HEIGHT 7 INCHES OR LESS	NA	NA	NA	•	
HANDRAILS ON BOTH SIDES	NA	NA	NA	•	•

ALLENTOWN PA	AMMAN JORDAN	AMSTERDAM NETH	ANCHORAGE AK	ANNABA ALGERIA	ARACAJU BRAZIL	ASHEVILLE NC	ATHENS GREECE	ATLANTA GA	AUCKLAND NEW ZEALAND	AUGUSTA GA	AUSTIN TX	BAHRAIN BAHRAIN	BAKERSFIELD CA	BALTIMORE MD	BANGOR ME	BASEL SWITZERLAND	BATON ROUGE LA	BELEM BRAZIL	BELO HORIZONTE BRAZIL	BINGHAMTON NY	BIRMINGHAM AL	BOA VISTA BRAZIL	BOMBAY INDIA	BOSTON MA
•	S	•			•		•			•	S	•	•		•			NA	NA		•			S
•		•		NA	•		•	NA	•	S	•	•		•	NA	NA			•			•		
•		•		NA	•		•		•	•	S	•	•		•	NA	NA			•		•	•	
•	•	•		NA	•	•	•		•	•	S	•	•		•	NA	NA	NA	•	•	•	•		
		•		NA						S					NA	NA	NA	•		S				
•		•	NA	•	NA	•	•	•	•	S	•	S	NA	•		•	•	•	•	•	NA	•	•	
•		•	•	•	NA	•		•	•	•	S	•	•		•	•	•	NA	•	•	•	•		
•		•		•		•	•		•			•		•	•	•		NA	•				•	
•	•	•		S		•	•		•		NA	•	•	•	•	•	•	•	NA	•	•	•	•	
•	•	NA	•	NA	S	•	•			•		NA	•	•		S	S	S	NA	•	S	•	S	
•	•	NA	•	NA		•	•	•	•	•		NA	•		•	•	•	•	•	•		•	S	
NA	•	•			•	•	•	•	NA	NA	•		S	•	•	•	•			•	S			
•	•	NA	•	NA			S	•	•	•		NA	•	NA	•	•	NA	NA	•		•	•		
•	•	NA	•	NA			•	•	•	•		NA	•	NA	•	•	NA	NA	•	•	•	•		
•	•	NA	•	NA						S	NA	NA	•	NA	•	NA	NA		•			•	S	
•	•	NA	•	NA	NA		NA		•	NA	NA	NA	•	NA	•	•	NA	NA		NA	NA	S		
•	•	NA	•	NA		•	•	•	•	NA	NA	•	NA	•	•	NA	NA	NA	•	•	•	•		
NA	NA	NA	NA	NA		•	NA		NA	•	NA	NA	NA	NA	NA	NA	NA	NA	NA	NA	NA	NA	NA	NA
NA	NA	NA	•	NA		•	NA	NA	•	•	NA	NA	NA	NA	•	NA	NA	NA	NA	NA	NA	NA	NA	NA
NA		NA		NA		•	•		NA	NA	•	NA	•	NA	•	NA	NA	NA	NA		•	NA		
•	•	•	•	•	•	•		•	•	•	•	•	•	•	•		•	•	•	•	•	•	•	•
•	•	•	S		•		S	•	•		•		•	•	•	•		•	•		•	•	•	S
•		•	•			•	•		•	•	•	NA	•	•	•		•	•		•	•		•	•
•	•	•	•	•	S	•	•	•	•	•	•	•	•	•	•	S	•	•	NA	•	•	•	•	•
•	•	•	•	•	NA	•	•	•	•	•	•	•	•	•	•	•	•	•	•	•	•	•	•	•
•	NA	•	•		NA		•	•		NA	NA		NA	•	•	•	NA	NA	•	NA	•			•
•	NA	•	•		NA		•	•	NA	NA	NA		NA	•	•	•	NA	NA		NA		NA	•	•
	NA	•	•		NA		•	•	NA	NA	NA		NA		•	•	NA	NA		NA		NA	•	S
•	NA	•	•		NA		•	•	NA	NA	NA		NA		•	NA	NA		NA		NA	•	•	
•	NA	•	•		NA		•	•	NA	NA	NA		NA		•	NA	NA		NA		NA	•	•	
•	NA		•		NA	S	S	NA	NA	NA		NA	•		•	NA	NA		NA		NA	•	S	
	NA		•		NA		•	NA	NA	NA		NA	•		•	NA	NA		NA		NA	•	S	
•	NA	•	•	NA	NA		S	•			NA	•		•		•			•	NA	•	•	•	
•	•	•	•	NA	NA	•		•		•	•	NA	•		•	•	•	•		•	NA	•	•	•
•	•	•	•	NA	NA	•	•	•	•	•	NA	•		•	•	•	•	•		•	NA	•	•	•
•	•	•	•	NA	NA	•	•	•	•	•	NA	•		•	•	•	•	•		•	NA	•	•	•

How To Use This Guide

Facilities for each airport terminal are listed on two facing pages: be sure to check columns listed under your terminal on **both** pages. A ruler, colored pencil or crayon can help align or highlight data in columns under each terminal.

as well as your local carrier, to find out what accommodations have been made. You might also request any literature that's available. For example, Greyhound publishes a small, free pamphlet called *A Helping Hand from Greyhound* (Greyhound Lines, Inc., 111 West Clarendon Avenue, Phoenix, AZ 85077). The booklet also tells you how to get a certificate of eligibility from your doctor so that your companion can travel free of charge.

The railroads have been a bit more of a problem in the past, mostly because the terminals and the boarding platforms were designed about the time of the Pony Express. Some changes have been made, notably in terminals such as Washington, D.C., but others still remain archaic and difficult to use. Amtrak also publishes a booklet that may be of help. It's called *Access Amtrak* (Amtrak, Office of Consumer Relations, 400 North Capitol Street, N.W., Washington, DC 20001). It's free, and it gives some suggestions for the questions you might want to ask about the particular train you're taking. For example:

- Will I be able to move unassisted from the street, through the station, to the train platform, and onto the train?

- Are there wheelchairs available at my stations?

- Will I need to bring an attendant?

- Are the aisles on the train wide enough for my wheelchair?

- I have difficulty walking through a moving train. Will someone be available to bring my meals to my seat or room?

Each scheduled train will bring different problems, of course, depending upon the kind of equipment being used. I read, with a smile, a little item in the bulletin put out by Flying Wheels Travel (see the list at the end of the chapter) in which Judd and Barbara Jacobson wrote:

> *Interested in a Chicago to Seattle route? Amtrak's new Superliner has an accessible entrance to every car! There is room for only one chair in each coach car, but we feel that one is better than none! Each coach car has an accessible wheelchair bathroom and they even have special wheelie units in the sleeping cars! That's the good news. The bad news is that you cannot wheel from car to car and*

therefore an attendant from the dining car would have to bring your meal to you—but maybe it's on a silver platter!

RENTAL CARS

All of the major car renters now offer hand-control cars at key destinations—Avis, Hertz, National, and Budget are included. As always, it takes preplanning and notification—information as to city, right- or left-handed drive controls, and how long you'll need the vehicle.

CRUISE SHIPS

This is probably the most difficult of travel methods for the disabled person who needs to use a wheelchair. The doorways of most ships are much too narrow to permit easy access, the passageways and stairways present an obstacle course that is almost impossible to overcome, staterooms are tiny, bathrooms also inaccessible, and there are bulkheads all over the ship that manage to block the wheelchair at every turn.

Travel agents who specialize in tours for the handicapped almost unanimously state that the only ship now fully equipped for the kind of access needed by the handicapped is the QE-2 of the Cunard Line. Other cruise lines do make an attempt to assist the handicapped, but the physical structure of the ship makes it a difficult trip for those who are in wheelchairs. Some ships are being refitted at great cost, but there is still no definite word that they will be any easier in terms of access. Check them out carefully before you even begin to book your trip.

As this was being written, I was filming my documentaries for Holland-America Cruises. Aboard our ships, I saw several wheelchair travelers and I checked out facilities myself. Most areas of today's ships provide access plus a specific number of rooms that can accommodate wheelchair travelers.

However, I decided that the best type of research would be achieved if I could get the information first-hand from someone who travels around the world in his wheelchair. So, with book deadlines waiting, Charles Gerras, my indomitable editor, sailed aboard the QE-2 with his wife, Anne, and here is his first-hand report: (It is also a perfect opportunity for the author to edit his editor's copy!)

Long live the Queen! Sailing the QE-2 would be a treat even if you had to use a stretcher to get around. In a wheelchair it's a breeze. Anyone who can manage in a modern hotel will have no trouble with this ship.

147

Think of it as a floating Hyatt House with spray coming from the waves instead of from the waterfalls.

Passageways are about as wide as the corridors in a hotel, and the same is true for the doorways to all of the public rooms. The dining rooms, lounges, bars, theater, and casino are all accessible, and on a level. Getting out on deck involves some tricky (but manageable) ramps, and once outside there is plenty of room to sit in the sun or in the shade at an umbrella table.

The QE-2 is longer than three football fields, and that adds up to plenty of huffing and puffing if you're pushing a wheelchair over those thick rugs. Therefore, it makes sense to book a cabin strategically located amidships; that way, you're always at least halfway to where you want to go. Our cabin (number 2090) was perfectly situated a few feet from the center bank of elevators which serviced every level of the ship. Also, this is the location that provides the smoothest ride.

Think about distances when you book your table in the dining room on this ship. Our table was clear across the room from the entrance to the enormous Columbia Restaurant. At first it seemed fine—a pleasant place to sit, and we had excellent service. But after a couple of days of wheeling through this very large dining room, over thick rugs and past bustling waiters during busy mealtimes, I resolved to get a table close to the entrance on my next cruise.

Getting the right cabin is critical. Price cannot be a major consideration. The cabin must be large enough to accommodate a wheelchair, and that means it will cost—plenty. Space is, after all, what you pay for on a ship, so chances are that a suitable cabin will have to be in the first class or the luxury category.

I checked out one of the lower-cost cabins (not the cheapest, by any means) and found that I couldn't get past the foot of the bed to go in. If I had been able to get in, I would have had no room to turn around to come out! In another cabin (a little more expensive), the bathroom was located at the end of a small dressing area, too narrow for the wheelchair to pass through. Our cabin presented no space problems, but it was expensive. You just can't go on the cheap here.

My one trouble was the bathroom entrance. Apparently, all ships' bathrooms have a bulkhead at the door—a metal lip about two inches high to contain any overflow water. There's no way to get a wheelchair over this barrier without help, unless you can stand or walk a few steps, of course. It's the one insurmountable element I ran into on the ship. I have no doubt that the room steward would gladly help with this (my wife helped me)—but, face it, it's awkward.

I've been asked if the motion of the ship presented any serious problems. The answer is no, provided you remember to compensate for it. Even the gentlest roll of the ship might catch you off balance at a critical moment. I was transferring from bed to chair when an unexpected, slight motion tipped me onto the floor. But after that, I was on the alert and that's all it takes.

I learned the Lesson of the Brakes one night when I was getting ready for bed. I was bent over, untying my shoelaces, when suddenly I saw the rug going by me at an alarming speed. I hastily applied my wheelchair brakes just as my head was about to crash into the dresser. Even an imperceptible roll of the ship creates an incline that can make a wheelchair travel! Put your brakes on when you want to stay put.

Would I cruise on the QE-2 again? In a minute! The QE-2 lives up to its billing as a wheelchair-accessible ship. If I can manage it, I'm sure just about any disabled person can. Those who can stand or walk some (as a paraplegic I can do neither) need have absolutely no concern. The crew is courteous and helpful, and the pampering they give to everyone is a rare experience in these times. I want more.

HOTELS

Charlie Gerras suggests that, no matter what your travel agent says, you have to check out the hotel for yourself. He recently went to Puerto Rico on a vacation and came back to report that he arrived at his hotel and found that there was no access for his wheelchair to most of the public rooms, the elevators were too narrow, and he began his vacation trip by having to find another hotel room in the midst of the high travel season. All this, even after assurances from his travel agent.

• Find out about steps leading to the hotel. If there are steps, is there a wheelchair entrance?

• What about steps to the elevators? After discussing this with Charlie, I realized that there are at least five of my favorite European hotels that have three or more steps leading to their elevators! Check out the steps to the dining room. Is there easy access for a wheelchair?

• The bathrooms are critical, of course. In most of them, you can't get the wheelchair close enough to the toilet; the height of the chair and the distance to the toilet make it an impossible move. There generally is no leverage at all, and certainly few handrails exist in the older buildings. Ask

149

for a ballroom chair or a sturdy armless chair of some type and transfer from the wheelchair at the door.

Some of the newer hotels and motels, and some of the refurbished ones, now have wheelchair accommodations. Others have a small number of rooms specially designed just for the physically disabled. In spite of what your travel agent says, check it out yourself. You will probably find that the larger chains, such as Holiday Inn, Hyatt, Best Western, Sheraton, Hilton, Marriott, all have made efforts to provide service in this area.

RESTAURANTS

Don't forget to call ahead and ask them if they can handle a wheelchair. And ask for a table that is large enough to accommodate your party—including the wheelchair—without your getting in the way of the bustling traffic.

SIGHT-SEEING

In the United States, the sight-seeing part of the trip is becoming easier, though it is no means completely solved. Most of the major attractions from Disney World to the national parks have made an effort on behalf of the wheelchair traveler and other disabled persons. Certainly, a part of it has been due to the growing market that they represent, but no small part is also due to the fact that new laws have been passed, and the government has been enforcing these laws to see to it that architectural barriers come down for the aged, the wheelchair traveler, the blind, and the deaf. In this area, too, pamphlets and publications are being turned out at an amazing rate by government agencies and by the tourist offices of foreign countries. For example, there is a publication available called *Access National Parks: A Guide for Handicapped Visitors* (U.S. Government Printing Office, Superintendent of Documents, Washington, DC 20402, Stock No. 024-005-00691-5, $3.50).

The British Tourist Authority publishes a pamphlet called *Britain for the Disabled* (free from the British Tourist Authority, 680 Fifth Avenue, New York, NY 10019, or from their branch offices in Chicago or Los Angeles). The Travel Division of the French government issues a guide for handicapped people who must use Orly Airport in Paris as a gateway *(Guide des Handicapés)*. It's in both English and French. In addition, you will find that the famous Michelin guidebooks have notations throughout indicating the accessibility of various places for the handicapped. (If you'd like even more detailed information, write to: Le Comité National Français de Liaison Pour la Réadaptation des Handicapés, 38 Boulevard Raspail, 75007 Paris, France. They publish pamphlets and books that give information about sight-seeing, hotels, restaurants, and shopping.)

The government of Israel also gives information, such as in their booklet *Access in Israel* (available from Rehabilitation World, 20 West Fortieth Street, New York, NY 10018). I cannot begin to be complete. What I am trying to say is that even a brief series of inquiries to the countries mentioned above has given me the beginnings of a seemingly endless list. Before you go, just contact the government travel division or the consulate of the destination country.

However, even with the information that I've suggested and the booklets you will discover for yourself, I still suggest that you check out sight-seeing problems, especially in Europe. The buildings are old, which is one of the reasons that you want to travel there in the first place. As Charlie told me when we spoke of the problem, "The buildings were built when no one had wheelchairs. If you couldn't get up and down steps, you just didn't go out of the house."

- The chances are that your best bet for seeing the important buildings, museums, and monuments of a country is to have a car and driver or a tour guide to take you there. The buses, most of them terribly crowded and inaccessible, are just not feasible—and the special tour buses are not equipped to handle the wheelchair passenger at each stop along the way when the group gets out to climb the church steps.

- Another way to make sure you see everything that you want to see is to book a group tour that is especially equipped to handle wheelchair travel.

SOME BOOKS TO READ

My small boat at Fire Island is called *Piccolo Mondo* ("small world" in Italian) and I have proven time and again that it was aptly named. When I was writing one of my earlier books (*Bread Winners,* Rodale Press, Emmaus, Pennsylvania, 1979), I was introduced to someone who turned out to be of great help in finding new bakers and new recipes across the country. As a writer, she had met a great many interesting people on her trips, and her suggestions turned out to be a gold mine of information. I can now return the favor and introduce her to you, since she has also written what I consider to be one of the best books on travel for the handicapped. Her name is Lois Reamy, and her book is called *Travelability: A Guide for the Physically Disabled Travelers in the United States* (Macmillan Publishing Company, New York, 1978). If you are physically disabled and you want to travel, I'd strongly suggest that you read it before you depart, for she has taken an entire book to expand on what I have tried to do in only a very few short pages.

Another book that you might try, though it is a bit more general in tone than Lois Reamy's book, is *Access to the World* by Louise Weiss (Chatham Square Press, New York, 1977). These two books, along with the steady flow of publications and the increasing number of travel agents who are becoming expert in this field, should give you a good start on your journey.

TRAVEL
ORGANIZATIONS

It would be wise to check out your travel agent before you make your plans. Though most agents have access to literature and research material dealing with travel for the handicapped, their experience is bound to be limited. Throughout the country, there are travel agencies that deal specifically with tours for people with physical disabilities. I may not have included all of them, and if I've left several out, it is not through lack of trying. After much research, the names that follow kept coming back over and over again, and I have personally contacted each one to see just what services were offered, what trips they've taken, and what areas of disability are their specialty.

Handy-Cap Horizons, Inc. 3250 East Loretta Drive, Indianapolis, IN 46227 (telephone: 317-784-5777). This organization, one of the oldest in the field, was founded by Ms. Dorothy Axsom and is still run by her. She and her staff have conducted tours all over the world for spastics, paraplegics, the deaf, and the blind. Their newsletters and publications are filled with photographs of wheelchair travelers in Alaska, Hawaii, and Europe.

Flying Wheels Travel Group. 143 West Bridge Street, Box 382, Owatonna, MN 55060 (telephone: 1-800-533-0363, toll-free). This one is run by Judd and Barbara Jacobson. Judd is, himself, a quadraplegic, and he's traveled all over the world with his groups. Flying Wheels services all categories of the physically disabled, unless the case is too severe. (They do not, by the way, run tours for the blind or the deaf.) Judd tells us that all arrangements can be made by telephone—there is no need to make a personal visit. Flying Wheels runs tours to Hawaii, to the Caribbean, to Europe, and all over the United States by motor coach.

Evergreen Travel Service. 19429 Forty-fourth Avenue West, Lynnwood, WA 98036 (telephone: 206-776-1184). Betty Hoffman, who is president and general manager of Evergreen, explained that the organization has three subdivisions: Wings on Wheels (for the physically handicapped), White Cane (for the blind), and Special Tours (for the mentally retarded). Mrs. Hoffman and Evergreen have been in business for over 20 years. She mentioned that, at the beginning, when she contacted the airlines about access for the handicapped, only *two* would cooperate—Western Airlines and *Iran Air!* However, more and more airlines and hotels are now involved in making facilities available. Evergreen has taken trips on African safaris, around the world, to the South Pacific, to Europe, and to the Orient.

Vagabond Tours of the Deaf. 611 South State Road 7 (441), Margate, FL 33063. This agency, run by David and Lillian Davidowitz, specializes in group tours for the deaf traveler. Their experience dates back almost 15 years. David wrote to me in his last letter:

> . . . *as a retired school teacher of the deaf who always had a love of travel since being a little kid, hitchhiking during the depression (once to the Chicago World's Fair when Sally Rand held forth), I traveled alone to Europe in 1965 to study the problems that deaf people have. I hitchhiked to Milan, Italy, with the Olympic deaf team . . . .*

He goes on to explain how difficult it was at first to arrange tours for the deaf, but gradually accommodations improved, guides were trained more thoroughly, and problems were eliminated bit by bit. For those who can hear, David's description of asking for services deserves its place in this chapter:

> *When I first went to Europe, I acted deaf and wrote in a Milan hotel that I wanted a room with a bath; it was 1965. He had to call three others before one could read my note. Europeans can speak and understand English but many of them cannot read it. Therefore many of the totally deaf would have problems and become frustrated in trying to make themselves understood.*

153

The group tours have eliminated much of the difficulty in providing service to the deaf traveler, and Vagabond has conducted successful cruises as well as trips abroad.

Rambling Tours. Box 1304, Hallandale, FL 33009 (telephone: 305-456-2161). Rambling is a family operation, run by Murray Fein, his wife Ruth, and their daughter Vicki. They handle tours only for the travelers who have their mobility impaired, and thus do not include the blind, the deaf, or the mentally retarded.

Interpret Tours. Part of Encino Travel Service, 16660 Ventura Boulevard, Encino, CA 91436 (telephone: 213-788-4118). This group is run by Ms. Ruth Skinner, who is deaf herself. They've been in business about 15 years and they've run tours around the world, to Israel, Egypt, Alaska, the Panama Canal, and the Caribbean.

There are over 35 million handicapped people in the United States, many of whom want to travel, many of whom do travel—alone or with a companion or with a group. The world is becoming more accessible, and the physically handicapped traveler an important and growing market to the travel industry. Eighteen years ago only two airlines would make arrangements for wheelchair patrons. Today, they all reflect the changing attitude toward people who were once referred to as "shut-ins." And the more you travel, the more the world will change to meet your needs. Bit by bit, the limitations and the barriers will drop, and bit by bit, the world will open even more. There are really very few places that you cannot visit today, very few places you cannot choose as a vacation destination—if you really want to go.

13

THE GREAT TOY FOOD REVOLUTION

With Unkind Words About Airline Catering,
the Ubiquitous Nondairy Creamers,
and What to Do About Them

There was a time in the travel industry when the airlines vied with one another to provide the most exquisite in-flight catering that the mind of man (or woman) could conceive. There were champagne flights, carts and trays covered with the lush produce of foreign lands, and—especially on the international carriers—a great talent hunt ensued to see who could snare the most famous French chef to design and prepare the airline menu. I remember the time that lunch or dinner on a transcontinental or overseas flight was something to be anticipated, a passing of the flight time in a most soothing and delightful way. Hors d'oeuvres of smoked salmon, fresh, crisp salads with dressings spooned from a bowl, imported wines from France and Italy, entrees prepared at Maxim's and rushed to Orly Airport in Paris to be put aboard the jet, desserts displayed in all their orange and chocolate glory to top off the feast. Well, actually, it wasn't really like that, but the airlines advertised that it *would* be that way and they did try. They certainly did try.

About five or six years ago it all began to change. Whether it happened at the same instant that America fell in love with "junk food," I do not know. But the airlines began to fall into deep financial trouble and the advertising no longer promised in-flight Utopia. We were not to be wined and dined, pampered and petted while on our way to a distant paradise. In fact, another row and then yet another row of seats was added to every plane, so that we now had a new closeness with our fellow passengers, knees crushed tightly against the back of the seat in front of us, elbows firmly planted in our seat-mate's noodle casserole.

The meals became smaller—and more inedible. Menus were selected on the basis of cost rather than quality, nutrition, balance, or eye appeal. An associate of mine, looking at the tiny portions crammed onto a plastic plate, began to call it "toy food." My dear grandmother would have said, "Pure poison—and such small portions." I could imagine the conversation between an airline executive and the caterers at Dobbs Houses or Marriott or any of the names emblazoned on the hearse-like boxes that lift up to the airplane galley and deliver that day's ingenious mixture of chemicals, food dyes, pre-fixed dinners, and nondairy creamers:

"I have only $2.10 to spend on each passenger flying from New York to Paris," the airline executive says.

"Oh, that's easy," the leering caterer answers. "For that we can give you one powdered egg, two small nitrate-filled frankfurters, a dehydrated pineapple core, and some instant coffee with a plastic stirrer."

The bargain is sealed and the meal will no doubt be placed in front of me on my very next trip. And I will not eat it. Either I will wait until I get to my destination to have my lunch (and in some places it may not be much better than the food served on the airline), or I will bring my own aboard. To that end, I will discuss in-the-air picnics later in this chapter.

I must hasten to add that I may not be alone in my distaste for airline food, for I have seen many others pass up the abstract collage of ingredients that the carriers call "dinner"—but I have also seen many devour the meal as if it were the ultimate experience in dining. I remember returning from Portugal, where some of the most pungent, aromatic espresso coffee is brewed. I overheard a passenger on the airplane comment as the instant coffee was served, "Now that's what I call real coffee—none of that awful European stuff!" To that gentleman, I humbly suggest that he skip to Chapter 14.

SPECIAL DIETS

For the rest of us—for those who must fly, who want to fly—there are some things worth knowing if you must eat the food aboard.

Special diet meals are available on most airlines. These can include kosher meals, light dietary selections, low-calorie courses, vegetarian meals, and an occasional choice of just a plain old sandwich in case you don't want to accept what they've selected for you. Sometimes these special meals are far superior to the regular fare. I have one friend who always orders the kosher meal, though he is not even Jewish, because he finds it's more carefully planned than the fixed menu.

Just keep in mind that the special meals must be ordered well in advance, usually a day or two before you begin your trip. On the other hand, there are times that the meal never does get aboard the plane in time, so it might be wise to have some snacks along with you in your carryon luggage. I remember a time a few years ago when I was on a low-cholesterol diet and I notified the airline of the fact. We were flying coast-to-coast and I had not yet learned to fend for myself by bringing food aboard the aircraft. As we took off, I leaned over to the flight attendant and smugly notified her, "Oh, by the way, that special meal that's aboard, that's probably for me." She looked at me, turned on her heel, and coolly answered, "Not on this flight it's not!" She and I talked later and it turned out that she really hated to fly and she didn't like leaving her boyfriend behind, since they were just engaged. Of course, I apologized for even thinking of asking for the special meal, and thereby ruining her trip, and I went off my diet with well-done beef and crushed potatoes.

(I realize that the airlines will excise this whole chapter, should they ever decide to recommend this book as a guide to easy going. But, in all fairness, I think they also know that not every flight is like the one they describe in the Sunday advertising.)

There was a time when almost all of the airlines proudly showed off their gleaming kitchens to visiting dignitaries and to filmmakers who were recording the image of the airline for posterity. Today, few of them have their own flight kitchens. It just became too costly. Nearly all airlines use central catering factories owned by corporations who buy their food, dehydrate it, reconstitute it, cook it with microwaves, ruin it with chemicals—all in huge batches on assembly lines.

One of the most startling machines that I've seen was in the catering kitchen at a large airport. Anyone in his right mind knows that chickens lay inefficiently shaped eggs. After all, if you slice a normal egg, my slice will not be the same size as your slice, especially if yours is taken from the end and

157

mine from the middle. Therefore, some electronic genius has invented a machine that strips the whites from the yolks, separates them into two large vats, crushes them, and puts them into a long machine. Out of the other end comes a long, sausage-shaped egg, the white placed neatly on a core of yolk, so that when it's sliced, every single piece is the same size. Each passenger gets the perfect egg slice on the salad plate! And, all of this is done within the parameters of cost-per-meal.

When you consider the gigantic size of some of these operations, and if you look at them as factories, not as kitchens, remember that machines do break down, and assembly line workers have an understandable inclination to let their minds wander. Therefore, it pays to be careful in some instances:

- If you're traveling in an area of intense heat, be careful of the ingredients that have a tendency to spoil quickly. Potato salad, salad dressings, mayonnaise are all potentially harmful. They can spoil quickly while waiting for a plane that is an hour or more late, and if they have not been refrigerated properly, the effects will probably hit you just as you arrive at your destination ready to see the town.

- The same holds true for flights where the catering is done at a stopover airport in an underdeveloped country, and the sanitary conditions in general are quite dismal. Why should the food put aboard your plane be any better? Because the airline is supervising? Ridiculous. The airline personnel at the stopover are generally indigenous to the country itself, and in many places there is a tendency to ignore the rules of hygiene— possibly including those that apply to your lunch.

- In other words, look carefully at where you are, where you have stopped, where the food has been put aboard. Pass up the things that can spoil easily—you are better off doing without the food than eating questionable ingredients and becoming violently ill. It has happened. I read about it in the newspapers all the time.

- These cautions apply for water and ice as well. What I say in a later chapter about these two potential poisons also holds true aboard the airlines traveling the lesser-developed parts of the globe. If you are uncertain, drink club soda with a squeezed lemon or lime and *without ice*. It will be warm, but you'll be safe. I have always felt that the unseen hands in an unseen kitchen, with food handled by someone who might even have a strong antagonism toward the Yankees aboard the aircraft, are not the best recommendation for the safety of a luncheon that is about to be served to me. I may be paranoid, but I do not get sick.

What I have written so far, of course, refers to the special trips that are too long, the flights that touch down at fly-ridden and mosquito-infested airports on five continents, the common-sense thinking that any traveler should do on any trip. But there is still another way—and, at times, it is a marvelous change from the routine and boredom of flying.

A PICNIC
IN THE SKY

There is no rule against bringing your own food aboard a plane. Liquor or wine is, of course, forbidden by law. But, along with your hand-carried luggage, a small picnic basket or brown paper bag or a package of fresh food can go through the security check with you and right aboard the plane. On particular trips, when shopping is available and where the food will not spoil on its way to the airport, I have begun to bring fresh fruit with me, cheese and whole grain bread, nicely wrapped pieces of delicious chicken, and even a few large paper napkins. The only thing that need concern you is choosing food that is not messy. It is difficult enough to maneuver in the child-sized seat without trying to juggle a bowl of homemade soup.

The movement has begun to grow. A strong ally is food critic and author Craig Claiborne, who has written several columns about airline picnics. And, in my own city of New York, small catering establishments, restaurants, and even a large department store have begun to prepare picnic baskets designed especially to be taken aboard the plane. There is a way to beat the system. Of course, it will cost a bit more than the $2.10 that the airlines are spending for your meal, but you will also be avoiding the scrambled nitrates on toast. Which brings me to another pet peeve of mine.

THE NONDAIRY
CREAMER

I have the most wonderful collection in my desk drawer. In fact, I may be the foremost collector of the item. While others collect stamps, matchbook covers, baseball cards, coins, gold, plates, or toy soldiers, I have the most comprehensive collection of nondairy creamer covers in the world!

I began noticing them several years ago, when the flight attendant made the trip up and down the aisle asking, "Coffee?" And then, "Cream and sugar?" I would nod, barely looking up from my copy of *Boy's Life*, and I remember being handed a small container. I abstractly peeled back the cover, thinking it was half-and-half (though I have never been able to determine just what the name really meant—half of what and half of what else?). Then I saw the label. The words were new to me, but I was to see them frequently after that. The label read: "For Your Coffee." It was, it said, especially prepared for the airline on which I was flying. Around the edge of the label were some tiny words, much too small to see without my glasses. Not only was I *not* drinking half-and-half—they had given me propylene glycol monostearate, di-potassium phosphate, hydrogenated palm kernel oil (and I was on a low-cholesterol diet!), and various other chemicals, colorings, and preservatives.

Fascinated, I began to collect the labels, slipping them away in a desk drawer until I finally took them out and realized that I had collected over 50 different labels in a period of five years of travel, each of them designed to prevent me from having real cream or milk in my coffee. They are a testament to man's creativity and ingenuity! The names are no doubt thought of in a late-night session at the nondairy creamer company with a high executive shouting, "Eureka, I've got it—we'll call it Flavor Charm!" (I have since discovered another more awful fact; many of the nondairy creamers are actually made by our largest dairy producers!)

And so Flavor Charm it is. And Flavorite and Café Blend, and Cup-a-Cream and Instantblend, Coffee Twin, Cafe Lite, Melloream, Coffee Whitener, Coffee Pal, Coffee Gem, Coffee Companion, Coffee Glow, and Coffee Swirl. The foreign airlines, not to be outdone by American know-how, have also introduced the nondairy creamer to their passengers. In my collection, I have two rare packets (which I will not trade)—Mikromel, made in Rotterdam, and Regilait, a product of our French friends. Some airlines are more honest than others, and the label merely reads "Nondairy Creamer." However, there is one that has always amazed me—it's called Coffee Coffee. It says nothing. It promises nothing. It gives nothing but more of the liquid plastic for my coffee.

But, as the public begins to accept all of this—under whatever guise can be invented (it keeps longer, doesn't spoil, the chemicals are harmless, easier to serve)—if it can get worse, it will. And it has.

Within the last few years, some airlines have begun to eliminate the liquid nondairy creamer. To replace it with real milk or cream—or even half-and-half? Of course not. To replace it with nondairy *powder* in a flat package. It still carries the same ingenious names, but now they can squeeze more of them on an aircraft already squeezed with uncomfortable passengers.

One poor old gentleman, sitting next to me, on the second flight of his life, became so confused by all of this that he totally ignored the packet of powdered cream (creme?) lying next to his cup and promptly emptied the container of salad dressing into his coffee. Thinking that this must be the way the airlines cater, he stirred it in until I whispered to him that the salad dressing was, indeed, not the cream (creme). He thanked me, called the flight attendant, and she replaced the cup, smiling reassuringly, "Don't worry, sir, people do that all the time!"

About three years ago, I found a way to fight back. Not only did I begin to take picnic lunches aboard the planes, but I also began to reject the nondairy creamer and to ask for milk—plain, ordinary, in-a-container, pasteurized milk from a cow. It is something that every airline carries and it's always aboard for the kids and for the sometimes-milk drinkers like me. Believe it or not, I have noticed it happening more and more. There are times when I reject the nondairy creamer and ask for milk, and then my seat-mate will do the same, followed by the person sitting near the window. (Remember that I always ask for an aisle seat.)

At first, the flight attendants seemed a bit annoyed, and, grudgingly, a container of milk would be put down beside me. Today, I find that the airlines usually keep an open container of milk right on the coffee tray—or, at the least, it's readily available to be passed from passenger to passenger who refuse to accept the substitutes. Flight attendants also report that the resistance is spreading rapidly. It is no longer unusual to get a request for real milk.

It is, overall, a difficult battle for those of us who have become aware that our diets were less than great all those years of growing up. I wonder. Is it just because I have become more aware of my diet that the airline catering seems so awful? I don't think so, and there are both good and bad signs on the horizon.

The bad? What I consider the final blow came just last week. The airline on which I was flying had eliminated the necessity of putting even a pseudo–toy food, rubberized dessert on the plane. When the time came to sit back and relax with something sweet enough to take the taste of the meat away, the attendants passed out ice cream sandwiches from a box—much the way the hawkers do at baseball games—tossing them to the passengers while moving down the aisles! This, I thought, was *really* luxury!

I opened the package, the sight of the vanilla ice cream sandwiched between two wafers took me back to my boyhood in the Bronx. Until I read the label!

WAFER INGREDIENTS: Enriched bleached flour, sugar, vegetable shortening (contains one or more of the following: partially hydrogenated soybean oil, palm oil, cottonseed oil), corn sugar, caramel color, cocoa, corn syrup, baking soda, salt, sodium acid pyrophosphate, artificial flavor, lecithin.

All that just to make a wafer? Was I now to begin collecting wafer wrappers and salt packets and pepper pourers? If the *wafer* contained all of that, what on earth was the ice cream made of? But there is also a good part, too. Somewhere up there, there is a culinary airline kitchen, a heaven where people are still trying. Not many, but *some*. Every once in a while, I am amazed to find that an airline meal is not only edible, it's downright delicious and well prepared. Frequently I discover this on the smaller carriers, the feeder lines with shorter routes, rather than on the larger airlines where the fantasy of their advertising quickly outstrips the reality of their food.

About two months ago, I was flying from Denver to St. Louis on Frontier Airlines, on a flight listed as a "snack" trip. To my astonishment, the "snack" was a full-blown lunch consisting of fresh shrimp in a scallop shell, a small, magnificently done steak, fresh tomato stuffed with fresh broccoli, artichoke hearts, and whole wheat rolls! I could not believe my eyes, for just the night before I had passed up an inedible canneloni on one of America's largest carriers, arrived in Denver too late to find an open restaurant, and was famished by the time I got to the airport the next day. I was, in fact, impressed enough to write a complimentary letter to the president of Frontier, for any encouragement toward more quality that I can give the airlines must eventually result in making my own traveling easier and more comfortable.

Possibly, then, there is a growing unhappiness with the toy food that the airlines serve. Possibly, the revolution against this abomination can really be helped by those of us who take picnics aboard and who refuse the little discourtesies of bored attendants and the lack of sensitivity of caterers who serve us the food that makes it easier for *them* rather than better for *us*. I can only say that if a revolution *is* beginning, I am ready to man the barricades. I have nothing to lose but my artificial flavor!

14

"HELLO, I'M HERE!"

. . . You Have Arrived — Some Introductory Tips . . .
How to Keep Cool in Warm Weather,
How to Stay Warm in Cold Weather . . .
and a Word About Altitude Adjustment

I remember our family's leaving New York in our Model A Ford to spend the summer in the Catskill Mountains. I don't think we had even unpacked the pots and pans and luggage that would supply us for the season (and how on earth did we ever get it all into a Model A along with a family of four?) before my mother had already taken out the laxative and shoved a spoonful of the awful chalky liquid down my throat and that of my younger brother. The explanation was, "You need it when you change the air!"

The summer would pass, and back to the city we would go, however reluctantly. Again, immediately upon arrival, after we had hauled the pots and pans and luggage up three flights of stairs, the blue bottle with the same chalky-white nauseous concoction was magically unpacked (I think my mother kept it right with her in her handbag), and once more we were saved from "a change of air." Luckily, I still do not believe in this ancient ritual, for I change the air so often these days that I would need a giant case of those blue bottles, and I'm afraid to think of where I would be spending a major amount of my travel time.

ON ARRIVAL

Mothers aside, the arrival at the final destination must be one of the great moments of everyone's travel life. Finally, we are here, whether we've made it up to the Catskills in our Model A, arrived at the national parks after a long trip, or landed at an airport where suddenly the air seems different (you have changed it, remember?) and the people speak a language that sounds like a cross between static and the backfiring of an automobile engine. There is a feeling of anticipation, of excitement, of the unknown—or, if we've been there before, a sensation of breathlessness at recognizing a familiar place. If we are leaning over the rail of a ship as it comes into a tropical harbor, we pick out the visual images that set the scene for us—the colorful houses on the waterfront, fishermen setting out in their small boats, or children diving into the placid lagoon. Even if the harbor is a sea of filth, we will still see it as a placid lagoon—and that is what travel is all about.

I suppose that the most important bit of advice that any traveler can give to another is to go abroad with an open mind. In most parts of the world, things will just not be the same as they are back home. There may be simple differences. For example, in Japan, the light switches, door handles, and faucets operate in opposite directions from the way they do in North America, and if you see a carpenter working, chances are the saws and planes will be manipulated by pulling rather than pushing as we do here. Cars are driven on the left in many countries, as you know, but more important, perhaps, is the fact that the drivers have different rules of the road all over the world (if one can call some of the mayhem "rules").

If you read your material before you left on the trip, if you are open and adventurous in your food habits (while still heeding the warnings about what you can and cannot eat), if you learn some of the language—even a few words—if, most important, you resist the attitude that you are about to "be taken" by every merchant, taxi driver, hotel clerk, and street peddler in the city, your arrrival will be one of discovery and enjoyment.

Certainly, the merchants in many (if not most) places just love to see the tourists arrive. They are, after all, business people, and the traveler represents a major source of income. But if they do "take" you for a few more dollars, what difference does it really make? How much did you spend to get there, how much does your hotel cost, what is the sense of losing your sleep and your cool over it?

I remember a trip to Saigon many years ago, and a walk through the incredible market in the downtown area. I spotted a woman who was selling an ingenious vegetable peeler, unlike any I had ever seen before. As the only

164

Caucasian in the market, I attracted a good amount of attention, and others gathered round while the bargain was made. I picked up the peeler, asked the price, and was told that it was the equivalent of 40 cents! The stares turned to me. I was expected to bargain. Possibly I could even have had it for 20 cents. I just could not do it. I wanted the peeler and the 40 cents were more important to the Vietnamese woman than they were to me. I paid her and walked off. Behind me the others giggled. The American had been "taken"—but what difference did it make? To this day, I take the peeler out of the kitchen drawer, hold it up, and say, "It cost me 40 cents!"

WHEN THE PLANE LANDS

But, I am already wandering through the town, visiting the markets, meeting the people, and I am, thus, ahead of my story. If I am to write a book about making travel easier, let's go back to the airplane as we arrive. (Ships are easier, cars still simpler.)

• Make sure you have all your travel documents with you—passport and visas—and keep them handy for presentation to the Customs and Health Officers. If the carrier has given you a landing card, make sure it's filled out long before you touch down. Have your international vaccination document available along with your passport.

• If you travel at all, you have noticed that many people jump up quickly, almost as soon as the plane touches down. Coats are collected from overhead racks, carryon luggage pulled from beneath the seat, children scooped up ready for deplaning. First of all, it's dangerous. There have been severe injuries aboard planes that have made a sudden turn on the way to the jetway. Keep your seat, and your seat belt fastened, until the plane comes to a stop. In any case, when everyone stands up in the aisle, it's going to take some time to disembark, and your luggage will probably take a long time in getting to the carousel anyway.

DAMAGED AND LOST LUGGAGE

• If there has been any damage to your bag, make certain you contact an airline agent or the baggage service people of that carrier *before*

165

you leave the area. Once you've left the airport, they will not honor your claim. If, heaven forbid, your bag did not arrive at all, or it missed the connection back in Denver, of course you will notify the agent, but I would also suggest getting the name of someone whom you can call later on to check to see if it was put on a later flight. Sometimes the airline will ask that *you* "pick it up later." You, in turn, will tell them to "deliver it to my hotel, please." Which they will. Then, keep calling them if you must, until you get an answer about your luggage. On overseas flights, of course, the "next" flight may not be until the next day or, in some cases, until two or three days later. That's one reason why I always suggest having an emergency toothbrush and even a soft sweater in your carryon luggage.

In Chapter 7, I spoke of the problem of jet lag. On your arrival, it all comes together and this is the place that it is bound to hit you. The first excitement will make you feel that you could walk the entire city and never stop. It is difficult to slow down, almost impossible to control your urge to do something, go somewhere, mingle in the marketplace. But, those of us who travel often have learned that this is just the time to take it easy, to gently discover the country.

AT THE HOTEL

• When you get to your hotel, unpack, take a hot bath or shower, and lie down for a rest. Remember the time back home rather than the hour of the day at your new city. Remember, too, that the jet lag will hit you within a few hours of arrival, if it hasn't already begun to work on your fuzzy brain. If you absolutely *must*—and it happens to me—just go downstairs and take a ten-minute walk around the block or down to the beach, then get back to your room and rest.

• When you do finally get out on your sight-seeing walks, take the hotel name, address, and phone number with you, especially if it's in a language that does not translate easily to English letters. Some good examples would be Japanese or Greek or Farsi. In that way, if you should wander too far, you can always show the slip of paper to a taxi driver.

TAXIS

Of course, you will have to read about just what taxis charge in that country, whether by meter or by bargaining, whether to take them only at the hotel rather than hailing them on the street, and how to tip the driver (or whether to tip at all). I remember the prime rule given to me when I made my first trip to Japan—don't step into the taxi unless the driver's eyes show recognition when you give the destination. Tokyo, for example, is one of the most difficult cities in the world in which to get around by yourself. When it was built, each structure was given a number depending upon its chronological construction date rather than through a numerical sequence. Thus, number 30 on a given street can be on one side of town, while number 32 can be seven miles away! In other cities, where the meter is supposedly used, taxi drivers have learned to tell visitors that "meter broken" (in any language, or even by sign language, you can understand it); thus the fare will be a flat rate, always higher than the meter rate.

• Make sure you know the neighborhoods into which you're walking. Some cities, though not many, are totally safe in every area. Since I mentioned Tokyo earlier, I might also add that the streets and parks are quite safe. In most other cities, it pays to ask the advice of your concierge at the hotel.

I will cover security in your hotel in a later chapter, but for now, the best advice that I can give is to carry your passport with you at all times. Leaving a passport in your hotel room invites trouble. Should it be stolen, you'll have to go through the whole mess of getting a new one from the American consulate or embassy, and it could well ruin your vacation. In addition, suppose you discover that it's missing and your plane leaves in about two hours!

DRIVING A CAR

Whether to rent a car is a decision that you will have to make for yourself, depending upon which country you're visiting, the rules of their particular roads, and how good a driver you are (or think you are). In many countries, it just doesn't pay. If you've never driven on the left side of the road, be very, very careful. Most accidents involving North Americans take place when an emergency occurs and the driver automatically pulls the car to the right, just as at home. Unfortunately, this throws you directly into the opposite lane of traffic.

There is another problem, incidentally, that occurs in countries where traffic keeps to the left. Pedestrians from North America are also quite vulnerable to accidental injury. The next time you cross a street, take note as to which way you turn your head to watch for traffic. To the right? Of course.

167

When you're crossing a street in London or in New Delhi or Nairobi and you look to the right, you will immediately be vulnerable to traffic coming from the opposite direction.

INTERNATIONAL ROAD SIGNS

In any case, if you do decide to rent a car and drive overseas, become familiar with the international road signs and symbols. They're quite easy, and it's puzzling to me that we have not adopted all of them for our own roads and highways. Even drivers with the intelligence of travel book authors can learn them quickly:

- Triangular signs denote danger, and the symbol inside the triangle tells the type of danger. This includes intersections, slippery roads, hills, and curves.

- Circular signs give the driver specific instructions, such as speed limits, parking regulations, and driving priorities.

- The square signs are informative; they tell the driver such things as where to park, the location of hospitals, and the proximity of filling stations.

Remember, too, that distance signs are usually given in kilometers rather than in miles (two exceptions are Great Britain and Ireland). An easy way to convert kilometers to miles is to divide by five and multiply that number by eight. A much easier way is to forget the *mileage* and just relax with kilometers. They're shorter, so they go by faster.

Gasoline is still more expensive abroad than it is here, so be prepared for prices that run as high as three dollars a gallon. (It is possible that gas will soon reach the same price here, at the rate it's climbing! At that point, the prices abroad will go up even further.) Of course, most foreign cars get better mileage than we do on our gas guzzlers, but you will still be appalled at the cost of fuel. On the other hand, if the country is an oil producer, you may be in for a different surprise. Last year, when I traveled to England, I paid nearly three

Opposite, international road signs

RIGHT
CURVE

MERGING
TRAFFIC

DOUBLE
CURVE

INTERSECTION

ROAD
NARROWS

PARKING

NO PARKING

TWO WAY
TRAFFIC

WATCH OUT
FOR CHILDREN

PEDESTRIAN
CROSSING

ANIMAL
CROSSING

TRAFFIC
SIGNALS AHEAD

SPEED
LIMIT

END OF
SPEED LIMIT

END OF
SPEED LIMIT

SLIPPERY
ROAD

DANGER

UNEVEN
ROAD

FALLING
ROCKS

NO ENTRY

NO RIGHT
TURN

NO U
TURNS

169

dollars a gallon; a month later, I was working in Ecuador where the price for premium fuel was 18 *cents* a gallon! (Of course, the cars in Ecuador cost three times that of European cars.)

Some gasoline prices are based on a liter rather than a gallon. And while 3.75 liters equals one U.S. gallon, I generally use a multiplication factor of four to determine what price I am paying for a gallon of gas.

THE INTERNATIONAL DRIVER'S LICENSE

You will need the correct license if you're going to drive your own car. In some countries, your home state license is sufficient. In other countries, you will need an international driving permit that carries your photograph and is only valid so long as your home state license is effective. Many countries are not signatories to the international agreement, and you may not be allowed to drive without special permission or a special permit. Check with your travel agent or the consulate if the name of the country does not appear on the standard international driving permit.

Though the major American oil companies have stations in some countries, your credit cards will probably not be honored. In other countries, the oil companies have been nationalized into one government corporation. Be prepared to pay cash (and learn the local words for "fill 'er up"), though on occasion you may see an American Express or Diner's Club symbol hanging at a service station.

GOING TROPICAL— THE HOT CLIMATES

Mad dogs and Englishmen go out in the mid-day sun . . .

I am, unfortunately, a traveler who suffers terribly in tropical areas, while I thrive when I am working in a cold climate. As the day in a hot spot progresses and the sun gets higher in the sky, I become more and more uncomfortable and I would like nothing more than to take my clothes off and lie still in a tub of ice. Nevertheless, my assignments constantly take me to the hottest places on earth, and I have learned to live with it by being careful, planning thoroughly, and "psyching" myself into a catatonic state when the heat seems to be getting too much for me. I cannot stand to be touched at times like this and my film crews stay far away from me. I am, to put it mildly, not the best companion in a tropical country.

Though the doctors tell me that perspiring is good for me (and it is), I once worked in Bangkok in the hottest season and watched in awe as my prize cotton shirt shredded into a thousand pieces while I was wearing it, the victim of nightly washings and floods of daily perspiration.

Others of my friends adore the heat, able to stay in the rays of the sun for hours while I crouch miserably under the too-narrow brim of a large hat and squint out at the hot, humid world into which I've been cast. For both of us — the heat-hater and the humidity-lover — travel in tropical countries can be uncomfortable at the least and dangerous at the worst. Over these years, I've learned what works for me, and it may well help you on your own trip to the hotter lands.

I am, first of all, a strong supporter of the natural fabrics, such as cotton. We live in a polyester world and, though we may look neater, the artificial, man-made, drip-dry fabrics are no boon to the traveler in a hot climate. We may look uncreased, but we probably are also more uncomfortable, for the very characteristics that make the fabrics "drip-dry" are the same ones that prevent the body from breathing properly and prevent the absorption of perspiration.

There's no doubt about the many conveniences inherent in the use of nylons, acrylics, dacrons, and all the other man-made fibers. They can be washed out in the bathroom at night, hung on the shower rack to dry overnight, and then worn again, fresh and neat, the next day. But they still do not breathe as cotton does. They only trap the perspiration against your body and, at the least, make you more uncomfortable. At worst, they can create the beginnings of prickly heat, exhaustion, fungus disease, and heat stroke.

It is no accident that the first observation that we make in a tropical country is that everything has slowed down. Our North American pace seems out of place, and it is. The normal workday usually begins at dawn, then slows down toward noon, takes a break for a long siesta, and then begins again late in the afternoon when it starts to get cooler. In many countries, the museums, the public and government buildings, the offices all slow to a crawl and then grind to a stop at lunchtime. The clothing is loose, sometimes only a long, flowing cotton gown for the women, loose-fitting shirts for the men, many times worn outside the trousers so that the air can circulate. Entire streets are shaded by overhangs, even in cities like Sydney, Australia, where the summer heat sometimes reaches well over 100°F and the sun shines constantly. The Spanish word *parasol* is literally translated as "for sun."

171

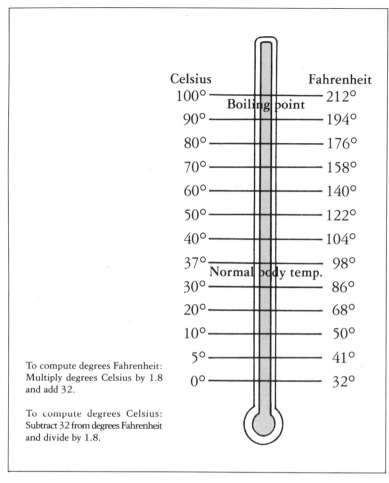

Celsius   Fahrenheit

100° — Boiling point — 212°

90° ———————— 194°

80° ———————— 176°

70° ———————— 158°

60° ———————— 140°

50° ———————— 122°

40° ———————— 104°

37° — Normal body temp. — 98°

30° ———————— 86°

20° ———————— 68°

10° ———————— 50°

5° ———————— 41°

0° ———————— 32°

To compute degrees Fahrenheit:
Multiply degrees Celsius by 1.8
and add 32.

To compute degrees Celsius:
Subtract 32 from degrees Fahrenheit
and divide by 1.8.

International temperature chart

Also remember that, all over the world, the temperature is given in degrees Celsius rather than degrees Fahrenheit. (And we, of course, are beginning to join the crowd.)

The best advice, then, is to take a good look at the natives of the country before you step out briskly to see the sights. The habits they've acquired for dealing with the heat are the result of long experience. The first reactions of some visitors is that the natives must all be lazy. Not at all; they must all be smart. The genial habit of a siesta after lunch is something you'll begin to miss when you return home. Generally, then, here are the things that will help to make you more comfortable in the hotter climes:

- Cotton clothing, of course — and loose-fitting, in addition. The looser the weave, the more comfortable you'll be.

- Light colors, since they reflect the light more effectively than darker ones. Among other things I am also known as a slob, but I still wear white in the tropics.

- A hat. *You must wear a hat.* It can be any kind, though a loose, light one with a wide brim is preferable. I have a huge collection of hats (along with my nondairy creamers), and I choose from them before I leave — a French colonial desert hat, one from Israel, another from Hong Kong, and a soft Amish straw hat from Lancaster County.

- Lightweight shoes, if possible, and socks or stockings made of cotton, never nylon. In some places I wear sandals, depending upon the sanitary conditions of the streets where I am about to walk. In any case, never go barefoot while sight-seeing — you'll be looking for trouble.

One of the things that seems to startle first-time travelers to tropical countries is the fact that it rains a great deal. The ads show sunshine all the time, but suddenly you arrive to find a veritable downpour. It stands to reason that if the trees are to remain as lush as they are, if the flowers are to continue to bloom richly and radiantly, then there must be some water out there somewhere. It does rain — sometimes it really pours — and you might arrive during the monsoon season or the typhoon season or the hurricane season. You will see rain as you've never seen it before!

Some years ago we were sent to Puerto Rico to film a golf tournament. Just as we arrived, so did Hurricane Jennifer (or whatever designation they had given it), and we sat in the hotel lobby for three days, watching the water rise and the crabs crawl across the floor until it was over. At the end of the third day, we also discovered that our camera equipment was covered with mold. The tournament was, of course, cancelled. All of this by way of telling you another bit of advice about your trips to the tropics: Bring a raincoat. However, make sure it's made of water-repellent material rather than a synthetic that is waterproof, so that it will not trap the heat and perspiration inside when you have to wear it.

Incidentally, as I go on, I find that I am describing the tropics as we generally imagine it. What I have written and all the advice that you will read elsewhere about heat and comfort also goes for the *dry,* hot climates. The desert areas, though they seem more comfortable because of low humidity, can also be as dangerous to the traveler who fails to take precautions. The reason you don't seem to perspire is that the atmosphere, being dry, is absorbing the moisture. Rest assured, your body is just as hot and working just as hard as in the tropical islands.

Take a shower daily, or even two or three times a day, to keep your body temperature down. Don't use ice-cold water—keep the water tepid or warm so that you don't shock the body. Warmer water also helps the capillaries to expand so that the heat will be more easily dissipated. (This also holds true if you plan to go swimming in the hottest part of the day. Diving from heat to cold can be dangerous.) After your shower, dust your body with an absorbent powder, and don't forget to dust between your toes to keep your feet dry.

I learned the trick of constant showering on my first trip to the Negev Desert in Israel, many years ago. The car given to us by our clients was, unfortunately, a *black* sedan—and though it had air conditioning, it couldn't work very effectively with the temperature soaring above 110°F and the black roof absorbing every heat wave in the Middle East. As a result, we took showers every time we stopped—at the homes of friends along the way, in hotels where we stopped for lunch, at a public swimming pool, wherever we could find the water. We took up to seven showers a day and they were our salvation.

Above all, make sure you maintain your fluids by drinking plenty of water (bottled in most places). Also speak to your doctor before you go, for advice about increasing the amount of salt in your diet. This is an era in which many of us are cutting down our intake of salt, because of hypertension. I personally have done so—I have heard enough about the results of high-salt diets in countries such as Japan to be forewarned. Nevertheless, this is one time that you will just have to ignore what you normally do at home.

The body needs salt to prevent the heat disorders that are so common in the hot countries. Whether you add more salt to your meals or you take salt tablets, the amount of salt necessary to sustain you in the tropics is almost double that of your normal intake at home. In any case, it is not a good idea to take salt indiscriminately. Ask your doctor, especially if you are on a low-salt diet or have been treated for a cardiovascular disease.

And finally, there is the question of sunburn. I have not forgotten it—and I know how many people in my own circle of friends like to return with visible proof that they were, indeed, in a tropical wonderland while I was slaving away in the cold, snow-blanketed Northeast. You will find more about it in Chapter

18. In the meantime, I will move on to talk about a climate in which I am much more comfortable.

KEEPING WARM — COLD WEATHER TRAVEL

There are times that the bitterly cold weather can catch the traveler by surprise. Not always for us the well-planned wardrobe that takes into account the vicissitudes of temperature or climate. There are the occasional surprises that make for the raucous and hilarious tales when we return home. My own experience in Sicily was one such prime example.

We had been working in Catania in the month of June. The weather was Italian balmy; warm breezes blew in from the ocean, and we worked in short-sleeve shirts most of the time. Through most of the filming, the awesome view of Mount Etna loomed over us, softly smoking from its still-active core. The temptation was too much for us, and one warm, summer day we drove up the winding road and took the cable car up to its final stop, then hiked to the top of the crater to film the view. We were, of course, neophytes, for Etna is 10,000 feet up and we started out in our summer clothing, feeling joyful and very warm.

Naturally, the higher we got, the colder it got. As we passed the barren fields of black, lava rock, and as the volcano drew nearer, the shivering became more violent. At the top, after the cable car ride, the cold was nearly unbearable and we were sorry that we had not remembered that the altitude would drop the temperature from over 90°F to about 35°F at the summit. Breathlessly, we rushed into the little shack that serves as both refreshment stand and souvenir shop, and there, before us, was a huge array of woolen mackinaws and warm hats being offered for rental. Obviously, we were not the only people who had forgotten how far the temperature can plummet at the top of a mountain. To this day, one of my favorite photographs is of the six of us dressed in ill-fitting jackets, woolen hats pulled tightly down around our ears, and the active volcano in in the background.

Of course, for those of you who are planning a trip to a cold climate, our fate will not befall you, since you will be deliberately including all sorts of winter gear. If it's your first trip to a ski resort or to a mountainous country in the winter, choose your clothing carefully and pay attention to the advice given for comfort and convenience.

175

Interestingly enough, the same theory that holds for hot weather is also the basis for cold weather dressing. Basically, it is the "layer" theory. If, in addition, you keep your layers fairly loose, the warm air will be trapped inside to keep you comfortable. The layer theory also works as a convenient method of doing a "strip tease." If the weather should turn warmer, you merely remove one layer of clothing, leaving the rest intact. You might "layer" yourself as follows:

- Thermal underwear. There are many varieties now on the market. I use the double-knitted kind—cotton on the inside, next to my skin, and wool on the outside. There are also thermal underwear sets made of waffle weave or a fishnet combination of cotton and wool.

- A wool turtleneck sweater covered by a shirt. Make sure the outer layer is loose enough to provide air space. Wear a pair of wool slacks with these, never tight jeans.

- A parka that is windproof and filled with goose down. Without doubt, the down jackets are the warmest, but you might want to try synthetic fillings because of cost, because they're nonallergenic, and because they do not lose their insulating properties when they're wet, as goose down will.

The layer theory can be applied with a variety of clothes—just so long as you remember that you'll get the most warmth by wearing cotton next to the body, then woolen outer garments under a down coat.

Use the same theory when you're choosing your gloves. Use a pair of woolen, cotton, or silk gloves topped by mittens, either fur-lined or down-filled. I have an excellent pair of sheepskin mittens that I use, and I have freedom of movement for my fingers, to prevent frostbite.

- Make sure that your shoes are not too tight, the most common reason for frostbitten toes. Allow enough room when you buy your shoes so that you can wear a pair of cotton socks under a pair of heavy woolen ones. You might consider getting insulated, waterproof boots with a felt liner.

- If you wear a hat in hot weather, you must certainly wear a hat in cold climates, albeit a different type of hat. There is tremendous heat loss through the top of your head, and though I am generally a hatless pedestrian during most of the year, I do make certain to wear a hat that covers my ears.

Depending upon where you are going and just how cold it's going to be, you might check with your local sporting goods store for the following items: face mask, woolen scarf, sun protection (the reflection from snow can be dangerous), and proper sunglasses.

I've also read with faint amusement the suggestion that you take out insurance if you're going skiing, just to cover the possibility of accident and the need for stretcher transportation back home! At least, I laughed at the idea until I did a film on skiing in Vail, Colorado, and watched in horror as the ski patrol made 20 round trips a day up and down the mountain to bring the accident victims back to the clinic and then to send them by ambulance to Denver. As a nonexerciser, you can imagine my dismay.

• In bitterly cold weather, try to keep moving to keep the circulation flowing. If you're a spectator at an outdoor event, such as skiing or skating or ice hockey, stamp your feet from time to time, wriggle your fingers and toes. If you begin to shiver too violently, get indoors, for shivering is the body's first warning that your body temperature is dropping too rapidly.

• Alcohol, nicotine from smoking, and caffeine will all affect the blood supply or the body temperature. Drink hot soup or cocoa or decaffeinated coffee instead.

• Above all, try to keep dry. Whether from the inside through perspiration or from the outside through snow or rain, the freezing will destroy any insulation you may have built up through the layers. It is another reason that those of us who work in cold weather recommend avoiding the man-made fibers. You should have cotton next to your body to absorb the perspiration, a water-resistant layer on the outside to prevent heat loss.

I will touch on the problems of frostbite in Chapter 18, but just keep in mind that proper clothing, proper attention to exercise, and an awareness of whether you are too hot or too cold can do much to avoid the problem altogether. And, since diabetics and people who have arthritis are particularly susceptible to the cold, it might be a good idea to check with your doctor before you leave.

HOW HIGH IS UP?
ADJUSTING TO
ALTITUDE

For today's traveler, "up" can be very high, starting with the moderately high cities like Mexico City, Nairobi, and Denver (all about one mile high), to Bogota, Colombia (about 9,000 feet), Cuzco, Peru (about 11,500 feet), and La Paz, Bolivia, the highest capital in the world, with an altitude over 12,000 feet in the city and 14,000 feet at their rarified airport, where you arrive.

The amount of oxygen in the air decreases as you climb higher, and though the cabin altitude of your jet may have been set between 5,000 and 7,000 feet, you were probably not active enough to have it make much difference. However, when you begin to walk, climb stairs, sightsee on hilly, winding streets, or try to run, you begin to feel the altitude. Should you be going to Mexico City, the reactions may be minimal, but arriving in places like Cuzco or La Paz can be uncomfortable at the least, and quite distressing if you react badly to the lack of oxygen. You feel a shortness of breath, a tightness across the chest, and, in some cases, a feeling of choking if the altitude is very high.

I have noticed that much of the travel literature either does not cover altitude adjustment or it is glossed over lightly. As with any other potential travel problem, the more you know about it, the easier it will be to adjust. At the lower altitudes, it merely takes a few days of common sense and of being smart enough to take it easy. From the moment you arrive, just slow down. If you feel fatigued, and you will, take a taxi back to the hotel. Eat lightly and go to bed early for those first few days. It takes as much as two or three weeks to become completely acclimated, and you will probably not be there that long, so you will have to compensate by slowing down your pace. You can just imagine what that means to some of us hyper types who come from fast-paced cities like New York. (This author, for the record, has a difficult time slowing down in any city.)

At the much higher altitudes, the problems can become more complex, especially if you do not adjust easily when oxygen is diminished. If you suffer from any ailment that might be affected by heights, such as cardiovascular or respiratory disease, make sure you see your doctor and discuss the advisability of visiting the city. And for everyone else, the advice given earlier is doubly important.

• Take it easy. From the moment you step off the plane, on your walk to the terminal building, checking through Customs—walk slowly, and sit down if you feel weak.

• Oxygen and medical assistance is usually available at every airport. Don't be afraid to ask for it if you feel that you cannot catch your breath.

• Take taxis and buses for your first few days of sight-seeing. Try not to walk too much. Eat lightly. Get plenty of rest, especially at the noontime siesta.

• The hotels in places like Cuzco and La Paz also have oxygen available for rental, and you can keep the cannister right in your room with you. The fee is nominal and if it makes you feel more secure, don't hesitate to ask for it.

I suppose that this is one of those places that travel books ignore potential problems because it makes the journey seem unsafe or uncomfortable. But I believe that any traveler should be forewarned and well prepared. The mountain cities are worth seeing—in fact, they are beautiful and breathtaking. The high plateau area of Bolivia that surrounds La Paz and goes as far as Lake Titicaca near Peru is an experience I shall never forget—but it is also at 14,000 feet above sea level. When we work there, we always carry oxygen in the camera car with us, and after a particularly strenuous hour of climbing and carrying and working, we stop to breathe the pure oxygen from the cannister. It helps, especially during the first few days of adjustment.

I have seen too many travelers forced to return to sea level within a few hours of arriving at the high cities, only because they were not prepared for the effects of altitude. So, take a deep breath and go. You will adjust, as I and many, many others have, if you use your common sense. Of that I have no doubt. A much more important question should be nagging you at this moment: Can you drink the water?

"CAN I DRINK THE WATER?"

... With an Additional Word About Ice

Of course, the article must have been describing current conditions in Mali or the southern tip of Paraguay or a small island in the Seychelles, right? Wrong! The news item went on to say that these outbreaks were occurring in California, Colorado, Oregon, and Pennsylvania! The symptoms are exactly those of the intestinal upsets that plague the traveler in the underdeveloped areas of the world—chronic diarrhea, abdominal cramps, severe weight loss, fatigue, and nausea.

SAFE AND UNSAFE WATER

I am not, by any means, advocating that you abstain from drinking the water in Los Angeles and Denver, as well as in the jungles of Ecuador. What I am merely trying to prove is that the water problem for the traveler is a very real one. Despite the macho claims and teasing of your friends who laugh and say, "I drink the water anywhere and I've never been sick," it is a bona fide consideration, especially in the lesser developed countries. I am also saying that good common sense is perhaps the most important attribute you can bring to the question. And there is no doubt that next to "Do you love me?" and "Where is the toilet?", the most common question ever asked around the world is "Can I drink the water?" To an approximate answer, this chapter is dedicated.

Just as the time-zone syndrome affects our bodies, so do many other things when we travel—change of diet, change of altitude, change of chemical content of water. In many civilized cities of the world, the water is, indeed, "safe" by chemical standards, and the population drinks it with impunity. But the traveler arriving in Paris may well drink the water only to be stricken on a plane on the way to Rome, ending up under a doctor's care when everyone else is out devouring the city. It has happened and it will continue to happen, mostly because the chemical changes often are just not accepted by the body. So we begin by assuming that even in the best of circumstances you can be stricken by "pure" or "good" or "safe" water. It goes downhill from there.

As you progress on your trip around the world, it is wise to assume that no water is safe to drink if it comes from the tap. I have seen the signs above the sink telling me that water is or is not potable. I have seen the little signs in the dining rooms telling me that the water is purified. I have been told by countless travelers and captains and concierges that the water is safe to drink. I do not believe anyone. I do not trust the signs and I assume that all water everywhere that is served in a city or a country where the marketplaces teem with flies and the sewage lies rotting at the sides of the gutter is totally, irrevocably unsafe. I make it a policy also to believe that the luxury hotel that sits as an oasis of Western civilization surrounded by the hillside *favellas* and barrios is no safer in terms of its water supply than the little newspaper-roofed shacks of the slums that slide down in the mud with every monsoon rain. Strong words, perhaps, and even a little harsh. But this attitude has worked successfully for me and for my crews for 35 years now, and there have been no real hardships as a result, no debilitating symptoms to plague us, few days lost from work or from sight-seeing. And, to top it off, we never really believe we are thirsty because we have found so many other ways to keep our liquid intake at a normal level.

SOME STRONG SUGGESTIONS

Whenever we travel, we add one additional item to our packing — a plastic bottle filled with water from the tap at home. It looks just like the little flasks that everyone was supposed to have carried during prohibition, and it always fits nicely in some small corner of our carryon bag. For the most part, we have never had to use it on a trip because we have been able to find substitutes for tap water, but I do remember one late-night arrival in Bombay, when no bottled water was available at that hour and we giggled as we brushed our teeth with New York water in a bathroom in India.

• For the most part, even in water declared as "safe" in the larger hotels, the chlorine content is still not sufficient to kill the parasitic organisms that cause giardiasis and amebiasis.

• Bottled water is generally available in almost every country in the world, but even this can be unsafe unless you have the bottle opened in front of you in a restaurant or it is brought to your room sealed and unopened by the waiter or chambermaid. Insist upon it! Travelers have brought back stories of urchins gleefully filling mineral water bottles for the hotels right from the city water supply. I, personally, have never seen it, but I do believe that it's been done; I always demand a sealed bottle of water at my table or in my room.

• Soft drinks, fruit juices, beer, and wine are generally safe to drink, even if the water is not. However, even soft drinks that use sugar may well be a source of infection if you're in the tropics, where there may be fly infestation at the source.

Up to this point, the rules seem simple, and they are. But now the complexities arise. Suppose that you have done what I suggest; you have not touched the tap water, have drunk only beer until you are quite bloated. Still you are stricken. It becomes a detective story. Possibly the cause had nothing to do with the drink, but was created by the *glass* from which you drank. The bottled water was pure, certainly, but the glass was just washed with tap water in the kitchen and it was damp when it was served to you. The bottle is sanitary, the wet glass becomes the villain! Wherever possible, drink with a straw immersed in the bottle (learn how to say it in the language of the country, or play charades by sipping loudly to the waiter), or drink directly from the bottle after wiping the top with a (dry) napkin.

Aha, you say—drink wine from a bottle? Beer with a straw? How terribly gauche! No, you can still use your wine glass or you can pour the beer into the glass that's put down in front of you, but make sure they're dry. Tea and coffee are generally safe at the better restaurants and hotels, if they've been brewed with boiled water.

Some years ago, I knew a man who had traveled extensively to the jungles of South America, up the Amazon, to buy alligator hides. He was an experienced traveler, a man of the world, an intrepid adventurer—*who always got sick on his trips.* One night, we sat talking about our travels and we began to analyze what he was doing—or not doing—that might be creating his problems. Finally, I asked the question, "Do you brush your teeth with the tap water?" The answer, of course, was "Yes." The problem was solved and his trips were no longer the adventures into dysentery that they had previously been.

Brushing your teeth with the tap water—if you cannot drink the water because it is not potable—is the surest way to come down with all the colorfully named digestive upsets around the world (Chapter 17). "But I only put the water in my mouth and I don't swallow," you protest. You do not have to. Just the mere touching of your lips is enough to do the job quite thoroughly.

- Brush your teeth with bottled mineral water, and wet your toothbrush in exactly the same way, using a dry glass.

- If bottled water is not available, use beer, carbonated drinks, anything but the tap water. I remember one rocky train trip in Mexico, brushing my teeth with foaming Coca-Cola. I may have looked like a mad dog frothing at the mouth, but I certainly was not going to use the water supply put aboard the train at the last village at which we stopped!

I remember another trip on which we were to film the Rio Carnival in Brazil, a joyous assignment if ever there was one. On the second morning, I bounded gleefully into my cameraman's room to find him, his assistant, and my electrician all stretched out across one bed, their faces green, their hands clutching their stomachs. It would have been humorous except that we had to be on location in half an hour. I remember giving them no sympathy while stating rather than asking, "You brushed your teeth with the tap water!" Three green heads nodded in unison. I must say that they worked that day anyway, but the job was not much fun for anyone on the crew.

For every traveler, I'm sure there are stories. It's just not wise to take a chance. At the least, the trip can be ruined. At worst, if amoebic dysentery strikes, it can upset your digestive system for the rest of your life. It doesn't pay to be macho here.

And while I'm at it, let me put one more myth to rest. There is a great belief, particularly among Western "civilized" travelers, that "the natives don't get it." Well, if it will make you feel any better (or worse), rest assured that the natives *do* get it! They suffer from parasitic diseases that are debilitating, life-threatening and, frequently, fatal. There are areas in this world of ours where children barely make it to their teens, and in some villages and slums three out of five die before the age of five. In many cases, it is the water and the sanitation that are the villains. Certainly, it is no reason to curtail your own travel or to change your plans. If I sound strident about the problem, it is because it does exist, and all the pooh-poohing and all the pretended ignorance will do nothing to mitigate it.

PURIFYING
YOUR OWN WATER

In most cases, you will never have to purify your own water. I have found bottled water (or beer or wine) available in some of the most isolated places in the world. But some campers, some travelers to the outlying areas may well have to purify their own supply. The U.S. Public Health Service suggests that you add two drops of 6 percent liquid chlorine bleach (the standard type that you can find in any supermarket or grocery store) to a quart of clear water, or four drops if the water is cloudy. Let it stand for 30 minutes. After that time, a slight chlorine odor should be detectable, but if it's not, add two more drops of chlorine and let the water stand for 15 minutes longer. One travel writer described the taste as that of "flat Scotch," but what difference does it make?

If you can't get the chlorine bleach, 2 percent tincture of iodine from your medicine cabinet, first-aid kit, or the local druggist in the village will do just as well. Add five drops to clear water, or ten drops to cloudy water (per quart) and let it stand for 30 minutes.

If neither one is available, you can also boil the water to purify it. Boil it vigorously for *ten minutes* or more, let it cool to room temperature, and do not add ice. The Public Health Service also suggests that you add a pinch of salt to improve the taste, or pour it from one clean container to another to aerate it.

AND ABOUT THE ICE

If brushing your teeth in tap water is a prime cause of dysentery, then using the local ice must certainly be second on the list. If you will not trust the tap water, and therefore you will not brush your teeth in it or drink it or let it touch your lips in any way, why would you use ice in your drink? Because "they" told you that it was pure, that "they" used bottled water in the kitchen to make it, that the hotel is the best in the country and it's a part of an international chain and they wouldn't dare make you sick. Oh no?

I remember traveling up country in Thailand one miserable, humid, unbearable day right after the monsoon had turned the country into a single bathtub of humidity. We were all thirsty and the warm beer we had brought with us had long since disappeared down our parched throats. We stopped at a small soft-drink stand, a thatched roof, open-sided oasis perched on stilts in the middle of the Chao Phraya River. I ordered a soft drink and my Thai friend, Saravit, suggested that it would be better with ice. I politely refused, but he persisted and showed me that the ice was there in sawdust, freshly delivered from a sanitary plant in Bangkok just that morning. It was pure, he insisted, and though I agreed politely, I still refused and began to drink the tepid soda from the bottle.

In the meantime, Saravit, realizing that he could never budge the stubborn Westerner, asked the owner to put some ice in his drink. The Thai shopkeeper smiled obligingly, took a sawdust-covered piece of ice from the large ceramic container and kneeled down to wash it off. The place he had chosen to wash it off was, of course, right in the muddy water of the river! Twenty yards upstream a man stood urinating in the same water! Of course, the ice was pure. It's just the river that was poisoned.

Essentially, you just don't know what is going on in the kitchen of a restaurant, of a hotel, or even in the home of a friend. It would be wiser to drink your beverages warm. And, as I mentioned quite strongly in a previous chapter, if the plane on which you're flying is serviced at an airport that might well fit into the category of an unsafe water supply, avoid the water and the ice during meal service (unless the water is bottled).

Just as I began this chapter with a story about the United States, I must also end with one, for there must be a moral in there somewhere. I, of course, think that my own country is the paragon of sanitation and good health. I have had a small share of minor upsets, but I assume that the water, the food, the ice are all good—even though some of the water in this country tastes like a chlorine bath. I spend nights in the motels along the road and I am awakened by the traveler who wends his way at midnight to loudly scoop ice from the machine that pours it out by the bucketful into a trough. Blindly, I had always assumed that this supply of ice must certainly be pure, must it not? It is being made in my own beloved country along my own beloved highways. I read with some amusement and some chagrin that this is not always entirely so.

The State of Tennessee has become one of the first to institute a new law to control the making of the ice in order to eliminate what state officials began to call "yellow ice." It seems that these very same troughs had become the repositories of various and sundry kinds of garbage thrown in by people who had some need to dispose of their unwanted items. Not the least of the problems was the use of the receptacles as urinals, generally by children who were on their way to or from the swimming pool of the motel! Thus, the designation "yellow ice."

I must admit one thing, though. I do travel through the thirsty parts of the world with equanimity and with a sense that I have been there before and that I know most of the rules. While on the trip, I do not have the feelings of being thirsty or of not having my parched throat quenched sufficiently enough to keep me comfortable. I get used to it, for other things are more important. Nevertheless, I find that the moment that I come home—back to my apartment in New York—I immediately run to the tap, draw a large glass of water into which I plunk about four cubes of ice, and I stand there, still unpacked, and drink it. And I drink another glass, and another, swishing the ice around to hear the cheerful tinkling of the cubes. However, if in the next few months you should read something about the water supply in my city, please do not send me the newspaper clipping!

16

THE EXQUISITE ADVENTURES OF FOOD

... But with Some Words of Warning About Choosing It—and a Few Gentle Complaints About Eating in America

I love to eat. And, as an amateur chef and baker, a part of the serendipity of travel for me is the discovery of new foods, new ways to prepare them, and the uncovering of little, out-of-the-way family restaurants where the dinner or lunch can be remembered long afterward.

It has been, to say the least, a memorable adventure. I have shared chapati breads with Pakistani fishermen in Karachi, eaten freshly grilled catfish from the rice paddies of the Philippines, tasted of the tender morsels of kid (young goat) turned on a spit over an open fire on an Argentinian pampa, hosted a ten-course traditional Japanese feast in Kyoto, acquired the recipes for the unparalleled crab dishes prepared in Vietnam. Each of them and all of them—and many more—have filled my travel world with joy. But each of them has been, above all, *safe* to eat. The world of food in travel can be an opening to new sensations or it can be another way to ruin your trip if you're not completely careful or don't use common sense. (Have you noticed how often "common sense" comes up in travel?) If "you are what you eat," then it goes doubly for the time that you are traveling abroad, especially in the countries where food preparation, hygiene, and sanitation are primitive.

Of course, throughout most of Europe, even in the outlying rural areas, food is not much of a problem to the traveler, though even here I have been quite careful from time to time, and usually with good reason. In fact, not too many years ago, two favorite cities in Europe—Lisbon and Rome—had an uncomfortable reputation for food poisoning due to fish, especially during the summer months. Most of the fish was delivered from sea to table in trucks that were either minimally refrigerated or not cooled at all. In Lisbon, particularly, the trucks came from the sea, waited two to three hours in the heat for the ferry to take them across the Tagus River to the city, and then delivered the catch to the restaurants. Since the new bridge has been built, I hasten to say that the situation has improved. But many an unwary traveler and many of my European friends were stricken. On the other hand, this kind of story is quite rare in Europe; the picturesque restaurants are very safe when we compare them to the rest of the world. I merely relate the story to prove that there is a suspicious part of me that always has small warning antennas out about food, no matter where I am and no matter how much I love to taste the native cooking.

HOW TO CHOOSE "SAFE" FOOD

In the undeveloped areas of the world, the rules get more complex, just as they do for water and ice. However, there are only a few important things to remember and once you've learned them, the principles hold true for any part of the world, on any continent, in any restaurant, at any marketplace.

The general rule of thumb by which I judge food is: "If it can't be peeled, boiled, or well done, avoid it." I remember speaking to a friend who had brought up two children while living in southern India for ten years. She laughed as she described the food problems, "The only things I think I didn't boil for those ten years were my children!" Once you learn to judge the menus at restaurants or to balance the risks in a marketplace, you'll find that you can still taste of the native cooking, and take back memories of superb seasonings and unusual dishes, while avoiding the perils that lie waiting for the unwary traveler.

- You may be, as I am, a lover of rare meat. On any trip to a suspect area, be sure to order meat well done. And the dish should be served hot. If you're in a marketplace or small restaurant and the lamb or beef is being roasted on a spit right in front of you, the chances are that it's a lot safer than what you'd get in some of the "better" hotels.

Much of the meat shipped to the cities in developing countries is delivered in trucks that are not refrigerated, and the same meat is generally slaughtered under conditions that might be considered less than sanitary. I can remember country after country in which I've seen cattle killed and dressed in the mud of a roadside village, from there to be shipped to the de-luxe hotel in the big city. Rare meat can be the cause of a slight bout of diarrhea or it can hide tapeworm and parasitic disease.

• Food that has been prepared a long time in advance is also to be avoided if possible. There are several reasons for this. First of all, custards, sauces, mayonnaise, dressings, pastries, cold luncheon meats are all subject to spoilage in hot weather. There have been thousands of cases of food poisoning at church picnics held right here in the United States because of food spoiling in hot sun. You can well imagine, then, the risks of trying the same dishes where sanitation is inadequate.

There is another reason to avoid cold, pre-prepared foods. The best of cooking, the safest of dishes, left out in the open for any length of time will probably be attacked by the swarms of local flies, many of which have been visiting the nearby fields of cow dung. I suppose that I have a tendency to write of this in the strongest terms. Yet I find that I peruse a menu in a restaurant and, like you, I see something that looks as if it will be the most exquisite of taste treats, and my tendency is to order it at once—then that little warning bell goes off in my head and, for some reason, I realize that the dish is a potential danger and I skip to the next item on the list. It's something that all of us should learn to do in about 80 percent of the countries of the world.

FRUITS AND VEGETABLES

• Fruit is completely safe almost everywhere you'll ever have to travel—*if* the skin is intact and you peel it yourself. You can eat it at the hotel, buy it at the market or from the dirtiest of fruit vendors. I remember my last trip to Ecuador when we stopped at a little stand in a tiny village and loaded the car with the dark green, juicy *cherimoyas* (custard apples), happily eating them all along the way to our destination.

• Keep some unpeeled local fruit in your hotel room. When you return each day, hot and tired, an orange can be both a drink and a quick source of renewed energy.

However, it's a good idea to avoid the lovely, colorful platters of fruit put out so often in tropical buffets. You have no idea of just when it was prepared, the sanitation of the kitchen, or the health of the workers. The "peeling" warning goes from bananas to grapes, from apples to oranges. Carry a small pocket knife with you as I do, and you'll be ready to try the fruit of the country anywhere you happen to come across it.

• The same thing that holds for fruit is also the rule for vegetables. They should be peeled and they should be cooked right before they are served to you.

Most food grown in South America, Asia, Central America, and Africa is fertilized with human waste. It makes for huge strawberries, to be sure, but it also causes a large percentage of the stomach upsets that plague the unwary wanderer.

• In many parts of the developing world, the seafood is quite safe — *if* it is fresh, *if* the restaurant or hotel is trustworthy, and *if* it is cooked well. Be especially careful of shellfish, since most of the waters in this world of ours are generously polluted. Never, never eat clams or oysters raw. They can be a prime cause of hepatitis.

The other word of warning that I gave earlier is the best advice for seafood. If the town or village is a long way from any body of water, if the weather is humid and torrid, it's smart to avoid seafood altogether, especially if the local cuisine uses sauces and seasonings that mask the telltale odors of not-too-fresh fish. Wait until you get to the seaside resorts.

For most of us who watch what we eat, a hot day filled with long hours of travel should be topped off with something light for lunch, and in the United States or Canada we frequently choose a salad plate. Beware of the same choice while you're traveling overseas, for tomatoes are unsafe unless peeled, and lettuce can be dangerous, even when dipped in chlorinated water (and have you tasted *anything* dipped in chlorine?). Not only is the salad itself a potential danger, but the dressings, especially mayonnaise, can and do spoil quickly. I strongly suggest that you avoid lettuce altogether and that you eat your tomatoes peeled and "undressed" in the tropics. You'll find, incidentally, that many good restaurants serve their tomatoes already peeled. If they don't, just peel them yourself right on your plate and leave the skins.

MILK AND
MILK PRODUCTS

Another source of potential trouble comes with milk, milk products, butter, and cheeses, since they are unpasteurized in most countries.

• Avoid the corner ice-cream seller, even though the idea of a cooling snack in the hot sun seems so very tempting. Even more to be avoided is the scraped ice dessert topped with multicolored sugar syrups. I consider them psychedelic poison.

• All milk and milk products should be boiled or used in cooking. I even avoid the little pitcher of milk placed on my table for my morning coffee. I drink the concoction black.

And finally, you'll be dining in restaurants for a good part of your trip. The kitchen is hidden, the workers less than careful, the menu questionable in part. You can begin by sticking to restaurants with good reputations, but the adventure will be missing for some of us if we only eat in the places recommended by our concierges. You can certainly be adventurous if you abide by the rules. One good way to tell if a restaurant is fairly clean is to check out the toilets (though I have been to some that don't even boast that simple amenity). If there is soap available, there are clean towels or paper towels, and running water, there is a good chance that the sanitation is above average.

As I write, however, the parenthetical comment above keeps coming back to make me smile—restaurants that don't even have a toilet on the premises. We, who are so used to clean restrooms on our highways and in our restaurants, are sometimes shocked to find that the toilet, if it exists, is nothing more than a thatched roof hut about 20 yards from the main room. And the hole in the floor is flanked by two tiles on which you place your feet, while the water (if it is there at all) is in an earthenware pitcher. These lovely "restrooms" are another reason that most of us carry a roll of toilet paper in our kits when we travel too far off the beaten path.

I remember traveling through Asia and hearing a story told over drinks (without ice) at the home of a friend who lived in Bombay. It's the story of the "left-handed cup," and each time I travel in the undeveloped and developing countries I am reminded of it.

The British colonials, ever fearful of the diseases that ran rampant through the continent during the mid-1800s, worked out a way to reduce the odds of contracting some dread infection because of bad sanitation and the problems of daily contact. They figured that there were more right-handed lepers than left-handed ones, and so each time they were handed a cup of tea they immediately switched it to the left hand and drank from the opposite side. It thus became known as "the left-handed cup." Statistical records at the Admiralty do not show if it really worked.

EVEN IN AMERICA

The first part of this chapter was, of course, devoted to the developing countries, while this section is, alas, devoted to a developed country that is slowly regressing into a cornucopia filled with chemicals, additives, and fast foods no different from the airline fare. And, as we travel, we find that the bounty of the land is no longer available to us.

Here, the problems are different. We checked into a little motel in South Carolina in the middle of the peach season. The grounds, in fact, were literally covered with peach trees, each of them bending under the weight of hundreds of golden-orange fruits, begging to be eaten. The idea of fresh peaches, ripe off the trees, is a picture that every traveler carries with him. The next morning, at breakfast, I ordered cold cereal with milk and "a fresh peach." The waitress looked at me as if I were slightly daft. Fresh peach? "Sir, we don't have any fresh fruit. We had bananas, but we ran out." Sadly, I ordered the cold cereal with skimmed milk, walked outside, picked a peach from the tree, and took it inside to slice it for my cereal. The waitress looked at it as though she'd never seen a fresh peach before!

Traveling through Pennsylvania Dutch country, the superb apple butter that is made there can never be found in the hotels in which we stay. Indiana raises some of the best duckling in the country, but menus there tell us that we are eating Long Island duck—and frozen at that! Jams and jellies and preserves and the lovely abundance of the country kitchens are now packaged in little plastic containers and left to stand on the table in all their unappetizing inelegance.

THE JUNK FOOD GENERATION

At least our travels through the undeveloped world can be an adventure in good eating, even with all the warnings, all the potential problems. The native cooking is at least a valid cuisine and the tastes are unusual and memorable. However, in this country we have regressed into a world of junk food, quick cooking, the worst of the "toy food" syndrome which I discussed in Chapter 13, on airline catering.

The bread is made of wet tissue paper, nondairy creamers are served in the heart of milk-cow country. The fresh fruits and vegetables are shipped out of the areas in which they're grown, so that even in Florida and California we are served "fresh-frozen" orange juice. One of the best books on the subject—one that makes me feel that I am not alone in my quest—is *The Taste of America* by John L. and Karen Hess (Penguin Books, New York, 1977). If you think *I* sound distraught about what is happening to the food of my beloved country, they are even more appalled. We are, indeed, the junk food capital of the world.

Of course, there is an obvious way to avoid a great many of the food pitfalls in this country—and in some countries overseas.

• The first way is to bypass the pseudo-French, pseudo-continental restaurants that abound throughout the land. It seems that every young couple who ever made a meal at home is now in business as Chez Vous or Cafe Coq au Vin. You are much better off trying to find good, simple, local food than you are in looking for the promises that just cannot be met. A fresh catfish dinner in the South, or good Texas barbecue served on waxed paper, or blue crabs on newspaper in the Chesapeake area are all better than the excuse that passes for continental cuisine in most areas of the country.

I remember traveling through Pascagoola, Mississippi, one night, and I stopped for gas at a local station. I asked the attendant where I might find the best local restaurant in town—one that served good, fresh seafood rather than pseudo-French. He pointed back behind the station and I looked carefully. All I could see was a dim doorway with a white and blue sign that said "Lew's." He assured me that it was the best. Every night about 2:00 A.M. Lew went out fishing, and every morning he brought his catch back to his restaurant and served it fresh and tasty to his customers. The attendant was right. The simple restaurant was run by Lew's family and the fish was as fresh and good as it could possibly be.

THE
ROADSIDE PICNIC

• The other suggestion is certainly not new to the hundreds of thousands of families we've seen on the roadside and in the parks who prepare or buy their own picnics. If you're in an area where the fruit is fresh and you can't get it at your hotel, you can certainly buy it and eat it near a lake or stream. A small, out-of-the-way bakery is certainly a better choice for bread than the assembly-line substitutes bought by the roadside restaurant.

Overseas, we have picnicked in France, in Italy, in Belgium, and in Yugoslavia, even though the restaurants were quite good and certainly quite safe. It was just a marvelous opportunity to sample local cheeses, fruits, meats, breads. The technique is simple. When you drive into a small town in the morning, watch the pedestrians—soon you'll notice that there is a long, thin line of people wending its way down the street with empty baskets, while another line seems to be coming from the opposite direction, their baskets loaded with produce, breads, and simply wrapped packages. Just follow the lines and you'll find the marketplace without trouble. The cheeses will have no names, the meats will glisten with temptation, and the breads will be crusty and golden brown.

Of course, you won't be able to do this everywhere. Most places will still offer the supermarket as the only choice. But, in towns like Lancaster, Pennsylvania, we have avoided our hotels to find our way to the market downtown at lunchtime, and all of us, the entire film crew working with me, have gone down the aisles and had our lunch from the stands that offer the best of the county's crops. In some places, "homemade" still means just that.

Alas, I wish I could say that our food choices are getting better. They are not. My search for whole grains, for nutritious food, for real food instead of chemicals gets more difficult all the time. Not too long ago, I came across the ultimate obscenity. The motel was set on a lovely river and it seemed to promise a quiet, restful breakfast on the sunny terrace overlooking the water. Of course, I could have guessed that the terrace would be closed to the public—and it was. I resigned myself to the dark dungeon inside.

"Do you have any hot cereal?" I asked.

The reply was to be expected. "Oatmeal," she answered.

Oatmeal is the only cereal ever discovered in America. Except for grits in the South, oatmeal exists in its own isolated omnipresent world. Someday I will, perhaps, be surprised. But I resigned myself to the inevitable. At least they had hot oatmeal.

"Well," I went on, "it's not that instant stuff, is it? I mean, it's bubbling on the stove the way my grandmother used to make it?"

She grew impatient with me. Too many questions so early in the morning.

"No sir," she answered rather testily. "It's in the refrigerator."

I winced. "Oatmeal—in the refrigerator? How do you heat it?"

"In the microwave oven, sir."

I ordered a toasted English muffin and covered it with artificial plastic grape jelly from an artificial plastic container, while I sat there silently and licked my wounds.

17

"AND IT SHALL BE CALLED MONTEZUMA'S REVENGE"

Some Facts, Some Fallacies, Some Information, and Some Tips About Traveler's Diarrhea

During World War II we called it "the G.I.s"; dating back even further than that, the British troops in Egypt prior to World War I dubbed it Gippy Tummy. Since then it has collected a colorful roster of descriptive terms, depending upon which part of the world you are visiting when it strikes: Rangoon Runs, Tokyo Trots, Karachi Stomach, Delhi Belly, the Green Apple (or Aztec) Two-Step, the Tourist Trots—or simply, traveler's diarrhea. The last two designations are probably the most accurate, since the greater percentage of victims are tourists and business people who travel overseas.

THE SYMPTOMS

Whatever you call it, the symptoms are generally the same—cramps,

196

nausea, severe headache, vomiting on occasion, and frequent visits to the nearest available (or not so available) toilet. The most distressing symptom, the constant diarrhea, can severely disrupt a trip for several days; I have heard a great many complaints from friends and acquaintances who "had a good time" but "got the touristas" on the second or third day.

HOW TO AVOID IT

At the outset, before I plunge into the sophisticated and numerous remedies recommended by everyone, including doctors, travelers, and the U.S. Public Health Service, let me hasten to say that there is one way to treat traveler's diarrhea in the most effective way—*simply avoid getting it in the first place!* To the accompaniment of sneers, catcalls, and boos, since you got it on the last trip and no sane person would deliberately set out to contract a case of "Revenge," you must understand that I am preaching *prevention* of the most basic sort when I give this advice.

The two preceding chapters were devoted to proper intake of water, selection of food, sanitation, good sense. If the rules are followed, if your head guides you in the serendipity of travel, there is a very good chance that you will never contract it at all—or, at the least, it will be a mild case due to change of eating habits for a short period of time.

All this talk of brushing your teeth in bottled water (or beer, if you must), of not using local ice, of choosing food carefully, of making sure that vegetables are peeled and cooked, meat well done, peeling fruit yourself—it works, it really does work. Our own travel record overseas with our film crews—in the most terrible places in the world—attests to the fact that the rules, when followed, can be very effective. We are no stronger nor weaker than anyone else who travels—a bit more used to the vagaries of the world, perhaps, but we do eat the same food, are subjected to the same water problems and the same sanitary conditions as our tourist neighbors. And yet, the number of work days lost for our film crews due to traveler's diarrhea is infinitesimal over the past 35 years.

THOSE WHOM IT
STRIKES MOST

In the same vein, it has been documented that the disorder strikes *young* people far more often than us older folk. The younger people have a tendency to ignore advice and, in some instances, *must* ignore it since their itineraries are frequently based on lack of funds, camping out, staying at the most economical of lodgings, and eating at the lower end of the restaurant scale. The older traveler, on the other hand, is probably a bit more experienced, takes better care of his or her health needs, and is more able to choose a trip that offers better accommodations and selection of food.

It can strike anywhere—and it does. Some time ago, a study was made of American student travelers in Europe; when the summer was over, it was found that 50 percent of them had suffered attacks of diarrhea at some point on their trip. The rate, incidentally, was almost twice as high for those traveling along the Mediterranean than it was for the students who had been studying or playing in the northern countries.

When we get to the tropical countries and to Latin America or Africa, the rate jumps considerably. American students in Mexico, for example, show an incidence of "tourista" that ranges from 25 percent to 35 percent within the first ten days of arrival! And this is closely matched by the traveler who visits Latin America for pleasure or for business.

There are various bacteria and other organisms that can cause the symptoms of traveler's diarrhea. Some of them are more virulent than a simple case of the Tourist Trots, and some of them, such as amoebic dysentery, may not strike the traveler until after the return trip home. Others carry esoteric names like *Shigella* and *salmonella* and *Giardia lamblia*. Not only do I not think of these names when I travel, I can't even *remember* them and I see no reason to awaken at night bathed in sweat while fearfully fighting off salmonella bugs. Suffice it to say that if you are stricken by traveler's diarrhea (even though you have followed all the advice I've given), and if it persists for more than a few days, see a doctor.

WHAT IT IS

I am certain (with no scientific proof) that many of the short-term cases are, indeed, caused by change of food, raw olive oil used in cooking, and even the stress of moving from city to city at too rapid a pace. However, on a more scientific basis, it has been discovered that up to 90 percent of the cases of traveler's diarrhea are due to a bacteria that we harbor in our own bodies almost from the day of birth—*Escherichia coli* (*E. coli* for short). Everyone all over the world has this bug in the intestinal tract. The only thing that distinguishes one from the other is that some *E. coli* are more virulent than others, especially in the hotter climates. Though we can tolerate our own through our own body's immunity, we fall victim to other strains if we come in contact with them. As dwellers in the intestines, *E. coli* are excreted in human waste and, following the logic of sanitary codes (or lack of them), you can easily see why the more toxic strains find their way into water supplies, food, and almost every object we touch. If a new *E. coli* strain reaches your intestine, it replaces the strain already there and sets up a toxin that affects the normal absorption activity of the organ. This results in all the unpleasant and uncomfortable symptoms of the infection.

If we think of our own *E. coli* as "good guys" and the other fellow's *E. coli* as "alien"—and if we remember that they multiply faster than rabbits in the tropics, and that bad sanitation only increases the risk—then the advice about *prevention* becomes even more important. I suggested earlier that you keep an orange or other fruit in your hotel room for your return at the end of the day. Good advice, to be sure. But suppose you have just returned from a small village, handled art objects at a native market, touched the dust and the grime of the buses and cars in which you've traveled all day. Then you peel the orange without washing and drying your hands first. You may fall victim to traveler's diarrhea and *you* will be the source of infection! Sanitation is really as much *your* responsibility as anyone else's. You should, in fact, wash and thoroughly dry your hands before eating in restaurants or in your hotel or in handling food of any kind before you eat it.

WHAT TO DO
ABOUT IT

If you think that I have been avoiding the question of how to handle traveler's diarrhea for these many pages, I suppose I have been guilty of rambling on for a very personal reason. Not only do I feel that prevention is better than treatment, but I also firmly believe that the attack of traveler's diarrhea is nature's way of ridding the body of unwanted organisms. After all, who wants the other guy's *E. coli* anyway? Most attacks are of short duration, and though they may be uncomfortable, the most important negative thing is that you are being dehydrated quickly; the fluids that are being lost must be replaced throughout the attack and for several days afterward.

- Don't eat solid foods until the symptoms seem to decrease. You probably won't even have an appetite anyway.

- Don't take drugs! If your doctor has specifically prescribed a drug (more on that later in this chapter), I would not argue the point. But I do feel that most cases can be treated without the use of drugs.

• Drink plenty of fluids. Fruit juices are especially good. Not only will they quench your thirst, but they will also replenish some of the nutrients that your body is losing through dehydration.

• When you feel up to returning to the hotel dining room, you can continue your intake of fluids with hot tea, more fruit juice, and even some hot chicken soup. Every country in the world has a version of chicken soup, and my grandmother was right—it works every time!

The U.S. Public Health Service strongly recommends the following formula for the treatment of diarrheal disease. The mixture reverses the salt imbalance caused by the dehydration, and replaces lost potassium and glucose. Take two ordinary glasses—dried thoroughly, of course:

In the First Glass

8 ounces of orange juice, apple juice, or other fruit juice
(This provides the potassium.)

½ teaspoon of honey or corn syrup
(This contains the glucose necessary for the absorption of the essential salts.)

1 pinch of table salt
(For sodium and chloride.)

In the Second Glass

8 ounces of carbonated water or boiled water

¼ teaspoon of baking soda
(For sodium bicarbonate.)

Drink alternately from each glass, supplementing the formula with carbonated beverages, boiled water, or hot tea—but avoid solid foods and milk until you are fully recovered. The U.S. Public Health Service also strongly recommends that infants continue to breast-feed, and that they be given plain boiled water in addition to the salt solutions.

AND ABOUT DRUGS

I have already mentioned the fact that in principle I am against the use of drugs, except in dire emergencies. I have nothing but admiration for the science that gave us antibiotics and aspirin. But I do think that we, as a people, tend to overuse them as well as to misuse them. My own family doctor agrees with me and, in discussing some of the drugs listed below, he advises against most of them. He also believes that the body does an adequate job of cleansing itself when diarrhea strikes, and that some of the antimotility drugs so loudly heralded over these past years can do more harm than good. His feelings and mine are supported by a great many studies. I strongly suggest that you discuss the use of these drugs with your own physician before you leave on your trip.

Doxycycline. This is a newer drug that is taken orally. If the *E. coli* responds to it, it can be effective in preventing traveler's diarrhea, if taken as usually prescribed—from the first day of the trip through the very end of it. In a study made of Peace Corps volunteers in Kenya and Morocco, it was effective for the three weeks of the dosage and for one week after it was stopped. There are some problems, of course, and some limitations. In some areas, the *E. coli* do not respond to it. Also, side effects such as extreme sensitivity to sunlight may occur. And it should not be taken by pregnant women or by children under eight years of age. For the latter, it may stain their teeth permanently. The individual decision as to the use of doxycycline must be made by you and your physician. He will have to consider your age, other illnesses, pregnancy status, ease of access to pure food and water, medical care availability, and whether or not the *E. coli* in the area responds to the drug.

Lomotil and Imodium. Both of these drugs slow the movement of the bowels and they may provide temporary relief, especially if you are also subject to cramps. However, they must be used with caution, particularly if the diarrhea continues for more than two or three days or there is a high fever or mucus or blood in the stools. There are diseases that are actually made worse by these two drugs.

Kaolin-pectin. This is the commonly known Kaopectate. It does nothing at all to help traveler's diarrhea, though the stool may seem to be altered somewhat.

Entero-Vioform. This should be avoided. At one time it was considered the prime form of treatment for the affliction, but subsequent tests have proven that it has severe side effects of neurologic damage if taken over a long period of time. What is more ironic, perhaps, is that it does nothing at all to cure the traveler's diarrhea!

Pepto-Bismol. (Yes, Pepto-Bismol!) Its chemical name is bismuth subsalicylate. Recent studies have shown that it may well be effective in treatment of the illness; however, it must be taken frequently and in large quantities in order to work. The researchers recommended from one to two ounces every 30 minutes—with a total of eight doses a day. This means that an eight-ounce bottle would be consumed each day and it might be impossible to carry enough with you for the entire trip, especially if your family or group includes four or five people. More important, perhaps, is the fact that the U.S. Public Health Service does not know the long-term effects of the drug when used in such large quantities.

And, of course, if the symptoms persist more than a few days, if you seem to be developing a fever, if you feel weak and unable to get around at all after even two days, if there is mucus or blood in the stool—it is time to summon a doctor. For most of us, however, the symptoms will disappear in a couple of days, as our own personal *E. coli* take over our intestinal tracts again. The feeling of malaise may stay with us for a little while longer, but the bout with Montezuma's Revenge will be over and the trip can be enjoyed. When you return, you will go over all the warnings again, trying to figure out what you did or did not do to make yourself a victim. The chances are that you may trace it back to one small moment of forgetfulness, one lapse in your normal attributes of common sense—or you may never discover the reasons at all.

Throughout this chapter I have been searching desperately for a story, for a funny story. Unfortunately, to the traveler stricken by the "touristas" there is nothing funny about it. I only hope your story can be told with humor after you are back home, and that it did not affect the trip too badly. Better still, I hope even more strongly that it does not strike you at all. ,

18

THE SEA, THE SUN, THE AIR, AND OTHER HEALTHY THINGS THAT CAN HURT YOU

Some Good Sense About Swimming, Sunburn, Jogging, the Heat, the Cold, and Auto Accidents...

———————•••———————

If anyone had cared to ask my mother about her rules for swimming, she would have answered simply: "Don't go swimming before July 4 and don't go swimming after Labor Day!" Anyone who dared go into the water before or after those dates would, of course, be subject to the dire consequences of pneumonia, chilblains, the ague, and a severe case of drowning due to stomach cramps. The fact that it was once 97°F on July 3 did not deter her from her firm declaration, "You can't go swimming—it's before July 4!"

Although I may laugh at it today, I must admit that if I'm on vacation during the winter or I'm visiting some tropical spot in mid-December, I still hear the echo of my mother's voice as I put my first toe in the water. For most

203

of us, swimming is part of the fun of travel. Today, with indoor pools as common as soda machines in our hotels, even in the dead of winter it's possible for us to finish work or sight-seeing or skiing and then run down for a dip in the body-temperature water, the steam rising to coat the glass that protects us from the snow outside. The pool, the ocean outside the hotel room in Hawaii or Fiji or the Virgin Gorda are always tempting and always inviting. We have a tendency to accept them as they are, placed there for our pleasure. As a result, there are times when we fail to realize that there are also potential hazards waiting for the unwary vacationer or business traveler.

Of course, the first thing that comes to mind is the star of the movie *Jaws*. There are, indeed, places in the world where sharks can be a threat to swimmers, and generally the tourist is warned sufficiently to be aware of the risk. Australia still has shark patrols on many of the beaches, and even on my own Fire Island on the Atlantic Coast I have seen the water cleared by the lifeguards while a sharply pointed fin slowly made its way through the water about a quarter mile from the swimmers. Florida has had attacks of bluefish while swimmers were in the water. These are normal hazards anywhere in the world and any wise swimmer will ask questions before going down to the deserted beaches that lie so temptingly outside your hotel window.

• In the tropical islands, beware of sharp coral. The colors of pink and rose and green and blue are marvelous to look at, but many of them carry dangerously sharp points and they can injure the unwary barefoot wader. They also can cause severe infections.

• I don't mean to sound like my mother again when I strongly suggest that you not swim in strange places that are unguarded and without adequate lifeguard supervision. I realize that the "good" swimmer will totally ignore me anyway. (We always had a theory that only the "good" swimmers went out far enough to drown!) I do feel, however, that your questions should include a quest for information about unusual tides, undertow, or other peculiarities indigenous to that area.

I think we are much more aware of the hazards in the ocean than we are about the problems that come with swimming in the lakes, streams, and ponds of some inland and coastal countries. Swimming in any contaminated water might result in eye, ear, or intestinal infections, particularly if you swim with your head in the water. When it comes to fresh water, the only really safe place to swim is in a pool that has been chlorinated. After all, if the water is not safe to drink, why on earth would it be safe to swim in?

In parts of Africa, South America, the Caribbean Islands, and East Asia, a particularly virulent parasite makes its home in the fresh-water ponds, lakes, and rivers. It's called *Schistosoma* and the disease (schistosomiasis) results in intestinal bladder and liver problems. Luckily, the parasite, which needs an intermediate snail host, cannot live in salt water, thus making it safe to swim in the oceans and lagoons that surround the countries in which the disease is prevalent (except for the aforementioned coral, tides, and sharks). So check carefully if you're in the tropics and the only place they offer for swimming is in a fresh-water pond or lake or in a suspicious canal. It's also a good idea to avoid going barefoot in these areas, whether indoors or outdoors. It is something that I have to keep reminding myself, since I love walking around without shoes. But there's no doubt that fungus infections and parasitic disease are also prevalent risks outside the water.

BEWARE THE SUN

Each time one of our employees returns from a tropical vacation, the badge of merit—a radiant, glowing, iridescent sunburn—is shown off proudly, accompanied by loud "oohs" and "aahs" from all assembled. I am not one of those who joins in the crowd of admirers, for I am a believer that the sun was made for apricots and not for people. In any crowd of onlookers or vacationers anywhere in the world, you will be able to pick me out because I am the one who is standing in the shade while everyone else lies stretched out burning in the sun. It is not only that I burn easily (which I do). I just firmly believe that the sun, however healthy it seems to make us look, is as damaging an invention of nature as the typhoon or the earthquake. At its very worst, the sun's rays age the skin prematurely, can change the pigmentation, dry out the skin; also, large doses of ultraviolet rays can be the preliminary cause of skin cancer.

Nevertheless, the average vacationer, with only two short weeks to acquire a tan, generally changes quickly into a bathing suit and rushes down to the pool to begin the roasting process. I am not the first travel writer to wince at the image, nor will I be the last. The literature abounds on the subject, the warnings are boldly displayed, the advice freely given—only to be ignored. How many times have you come down to the dining room at a tropical resort at dinnertime, only to see countless fellow-guests painfully making their way to their tables, shoulders red, faces scorched. You wonder just how well they'll be sleeping that night. And so, even if I am not the first, let me join the multitude in giving some advice, however much it will be ignored.

- Take it easy at first. The tropical sun is much more intense and, as a result, much more damaging to the skin than the rays in the temperate zones.

- The sun at high altitudes is also stronger than at sea level.

- Even if it's cloudy, the ultraviolet rays can damage your skin. Some of the worst tropical burns are acquired when the sky is overcast, mostly because the victim is unaware that a burn is still possible, and less precaution is taken.

There is no doubt that people with fair skin will tend to burn more quickly than those of us who have a darker complexion, but this very fact presents another hazard of which we are mostly unaware or misinformed. The fair skin will *show* the burn more quickly and more easily, but dark-skinned people are just as prone to the harmful effects of the ultraviolet rays as anyone else. I will never forget the painful tale of a friend of mine who is black. He and his family vacationed in Jamaica and thought that because they were black they would not be susceptible to problems with the sun. How very wrong they were! The entire family came back telling the tale of the first three days of pain due to sunburn.

- If you have any skin condition, or if you are taking drugs or medication, check with your doctor before you leave home. There are certain drugs, such as some antibiotics, diuretics, and tranquilizers that tend to intensify the effect of the sun. This also goes for some antidiabetic medication.

SUNSCREENS AND SUNBLOCKS

There are many of us (myself included) who dislike the feeling of lotions and creams on our skin, especially if they have a tendency to be oily or greasy. Just keep in mind, however, that if you try to avoid the sun by wearing light clothing and covering your head, you can also get a reflective burn that can be quite as dangerous and intense as that from rays from the direct sun. Sand, water, white walls—all reflect the sun's rays. The best suggestion is to use a sunblock or sunscreen to cut the dangerous ultraviolet rays. Basically, those rays fall into two categories: those that burn the skin and those that tan.

• To block both burning rays and tanning rays, if you have a sensitive skin as I do, choose a compound that contains zinc or titanium. These compounds are excellent, too, for spot application on particularly sensitive areas of the face, such as the bridge of the nose. They are exactly what your local lifeguards are using when you see those white spots on their faces as they sit in the sun atop their towers. These sunblocks are also excellent for those who might have skin conditions such as lupus.

• For screening and burning rays while still allowing a suntan to get through (so you can show off when you get home), para-aminobenzoic acid, commonly listed on labels as PABA, is fairly effective. The manufacturers and drug companies have developed a code that rates the PABA content from 1 to 15. The higher the number, the larger the content of PABA and thus the more effective the compound.

Whatever you use, sunblock or sunscreen, apply it *before* you leave your room to go down to the pool or beach. By the time you get to the water, spread out on your towel, chat with your neighbor, and finally apply the cream or lotion, you will have been thoroughly exposed to the tropical sun already, and your burn is well on its way.

• In spite of what the labels say, most sunscreens and sunblocks will wash off after you've been swimming. And, if the water doesn't do the job, the drying off process with a large towel will certainly deplete the protection. After you've been swimming, apply the lotion or cream again.

If you do get a bad burn in spite of warnings, common sense (or lack of it), or having missed reading this chapter and the thousand and one articles on the subject, the milder symptoms will generally last only a few hours or a day or so at most. However, I can only hope that your precautions prevent you from ever getting a severe case of sunburn that can lead to swollen skin and blistering. If it reaches that stage, there is a good chance that you will also have a beautiful headache, nausea, possible high fever, and you certainly won't feel very comfortable when you put your clothing on over the more tender parts of your body.

What do you do about it? Well, the simple remedies for the milder cases include slathering the affected parts with a cooling agent like sour cream or yogurt, or dabbing with a sopping wet teabag. For more severe cases, of course, you'll have to see a doctor. But once more, it comes down to the easy way to treat sunburn—avoid getting it altogether. Just as in the matter of food and water, the strongest advice that anyone can give is to *prevent* it.

FOR HIKERS AND JOGGERS

I, for one, cannot stand to look at anyone in pain, and I must admit that I wince when the joggers go by my walk on the island, panting and groaning like an obscene phone call. Nevertheless, I am liberal enough to understand that some people do like it and, to pay for my sins, I have just completed a short film about jogging and running as a sport and recreation. Many travelers take their jogging right along with them, of course, since the equipment needed is minimal and easy to pack. Whether you are just hiking through a new country or you are a runner who must practice every morning, rain or shine, mountain or desert, there are just a few short words of advice that this nonrunner can give to you.

• Beware of heat, beware of altitude. The warnings that were given in Chapter 14 go doubly for people who are very active while on their trips. Prickly heat, heat exhaustion, heat cramps are all hazards in tropical or desert areas, especially for people who exercise intensely.

• Take some kind of foot powder along with you, especially one that is effective as an antimycosis (fungus) agent.

THE PERILS OF HEAT

I've given some information about dressing for hot climates, but the active person may well feel symptoms over and above the mild discomfort that comes with just being hot. Watch out for exercise during the noon hours, when the sun is at its highest point. Tennis, jogging, and other exercise should be kept for the cooler morning or late afternoon hours. Now many resorts offer night tennis on floodlit courts—worth considering if you can't get a court at a time when the temperature is kind during the day.

One of the best pieces of information that I've seen on the subject is the IAMAT pamphlet (see Chapter 20 for address) *How to Adjust to the Heat.* Many of my own travel habits come from their suggestions on dressing for various climates, immunization requirements, and warnings about food and water. Briefly, though, the dangers are:

Heat Exhaustion. Generally a result of high temperatures combined with excessive activity—consider the rapid pace of today's traveler through nine countries in as many days. The victim should be taken out of the sun, made to rest, and be given salt and fluids.

Heat Cramps. An advanced stage of dehydration, common in hot and dry equatorial countries when the humidity is low and the victim is unaware of the need for fluids. The best course, again, is prevention. When you're in a hot, dry climate, make sure you drink plenty of fluids, increase your salt intake, avoid exposure to the sun, and get plenty of sleep.

Heat Stroke. A condition that can affect anyone—the traveler, someone who works in the sun constantly, the sports enthusiast playing in the outdoors in a tropical climate. It's commonly called "sunstroke," and the victim cannot lose body heat because of the high temperature and high humidity that makes evaporation impossible. The skin becomes dry, the temperature goes up, there is disorientation and delerium, and, in the worst cases, the patient may go into a coma. Again, the victim should be taken to a cool environment and the temperature brought down quickly by placing cold, wet towels all over the body.

AND ABOUT COLD

After all the talk of heat and the tropics, the perspiration and the exhaustion, let's move to the cold climates for a moment and remember our skiing friends and the hikers who love to challenge Mount Everest (or a reasonable facsimile thereof).

Here, too, the rule is basically that of prevention. Proper clothing, awareness of the dangers of exposure to cold, and knowing the warning signs of frostbite are the places to begin.

Frostbite. A feeling of cold at first, followed by a burning sensation— these are the first symptoms that frostbite may be occurring. The danger point is the burning, for after that the area becomes numb and you'll feel nothing at all in the affected part. The skin will turn whitish or blue. Get out of the cold area if possible and warm that part of the body with warm—not hot!—water. In a dire emergency, you can use urine to warm the injured part. Don't rub the injured part with snow. And if you're with your children, watch them carefully, since they are generally not aware of just when the burning turns to numbness and it is after this point that most of the damage can occur.

SOME OTHER RISKS

Actually, all that has preceded this can be read and probably disregarded on most of your trips. For many of us, the travel will be through temperate climates, with the amenities of civilization at our fingertips, warmed or cooled buses and cars, swimming in filtered, chlorinated, constantly flowing pools or on pure white, freshly raked, sandy beaches outside luxury hotels. It may or may not surprise you to learn, then, that the major cause of disability and death for travelers is not the purity of swimming water, the infections so prevalent in developing countries, or heat exhaustion due to climbing the Pyramids. The leader of that dubious list of disasters is—accidents! Automobile accidents lead the slate, and most of them result from unfamiliarity with local conditions, bad roads, unmarked highways, and less-than-careful other drivers. It's wise to avoid unnecessary nighttime driving, especially if you're coming back to your hotel after a night of celebration and even a mild intake of alcohol.

The final word of caution, then, might well be to take a taxi back home, but I must admit that I have also seen the worst of taxi drivers in this world of ours. Many of them made me feel that perhaps I *should* have driven myself!

I remember taking my own advice one night in Taiwan and, since I was to attend a party in an unfamiliar part of Taipei, I decided to take a taxi both ways. The trip to my friend's home was uneventful, but the return trip was quite memorable, if for all the wrong reasons. The city was deserted and the driver made his way through the streets as though he were qualifying for Le Mans—screeching around corners, driving through "stop" signs. I tried to slow him down, but he spoke no English and I spoke no Chinese, a distinct flaw in international communications. Finally, after a harrowing 20 minutes, I spied my hotel atop the next hill and breathed a sigh of relief as we drifted to a stop. The driver excitedly motioned, pointed, and screamed at me in his own tongue as the doorman opened the taxi door and helped me out. I paid the fare to the gesticulating, hysterical driver and watched as he rolled *backwards* down the driveway.

"What was he trying to tell me?" I asked the doorman. "He seemed to want me out of there quickly."

"Yes sir," he answered. "He was trying to tell you to hurry out because his car has no brakes!"

19

THE CREEPY-CRAWLIES AND AIRBORNE PESTS

About the Insect World—with an Added Word About the Anopheles Mosquito

It was summer and we were visiting the lake region of Italy on one of our film trips. The little hotel was in Sirmione on Lake Garda and our small, lovely room looked out over the water and the boats. Nothing could spoil the idyllic feeling of my beloved Italy, nothing could happen to spoil the perfect day. And so, we called the crew together and went downstairs to have dinner by the lake. The night was warm and so we left the windows open and the table lamp on. Both were mistakes, of course.

When we returned several hours later, sated with fine Northern cooking and a carafe of the local wine, we opened the door to a vision out of a Hollywood horror movie entitled *The Bugs of Sirmione.* The room was filled, literally filled—across the walls, on the beds, over the floor, flying everywhere—with little black insects. There must have been two million in what was once a charming, quiet room on a lakefront. I ran down to the concierge, asked for a can of insect spray and ran hurriedly back to shut the windows and spray the room thoroughly. Quickly, I shut the door and left for a few minutes to let the spray do its work.

When I returned, the job was done. The insects, all of them, were dead. But now they were piled one inch thick on the floor, on the clean bed, on the clothing, in the water glasses, the sink, the open suitcase on the chair, and atop the guidebook for the lake region of Italy. The cleanup took two and a half hours and I never forgot the lesson.

If the above story could happen in Italy, just imagine the results in some jungle area where the insect population is more aggressive and much more dangerous. Of course, we all react quite differently to them. Some of us scream rather loudly at the more repulsive-looking varieties. Others have learned to ignore them. I don't think we will ever really learn to live side by side with them and, if you believe that the insect population will eventually take over the world, make way for them, for they are everywhere we care to look, especially in the tropical and underdeveloped areas of the world. Mostly, the insects are simply a nuisance or a minor discomfort, but in many places they are the prime transmitters of infectious disease. I remember driving through Tsavo National Park in Kenya and suddenly the driver shouted, "Tsetse fly!" I will never forget how one tiny cross-winged insect could make five grown people move so quickly. We brushed it out of the half-open window as quickly as we could. After all, not every tsetse fly gives its victim sleeping sickness, but there's no time to find out if that *particular* one is infected.

INSECT SPRAYS

I must add a parenthetical word here. What follows is a strong suggestion that we protect ourselves with insect sprays and chemicals. I am well aware that many people are totally against the use of sprays, insecticides, and chemicals, while others will use them only when absolutely necessary. However, there are times that the philosophy of abstinence can be downright dangerous to the traveler; the potential of malaria or sleeping sickness can be very real and very threatening, while the discomfort alone of jungle mosquitoes can make life unbearable. It is with these thoughts in mind that I make the following suggestions.

TRAVELING IN
INSECT COUNTRY

For the normal, average, everyday insect such as the common mosquito or housefly, the precautions are simple. Whether you are at the beach in the United States or overseas during the summer months, the basic preventive measures of a good insect spray and a repellent that you can apply to your exposed skin areas will generally do the job quite well. When you get to the tropical areas, the simple rules must be followed even more completely, and, added to them, be aware of some other warnings given by the experts:

• Make sure you have an effective insect spray in your room. If you have not brought one with you, ask for it at your hotel or shop for it at a local store. Most insect-infested countries will have them available somewhere.

• Spray your room before leaving it in the evening. Keep the doors and windows tightly closed after the spraying, and turn off the light! (I know someone in Sirmione who failed to do this. . . .)

• Wear protective clothing and use an insect repellent to cover the unprotected parts of your body—backs of hands, face, neck, behind the ears. Read the directions carefully and notice how long the effect will last. Renew the application whenever necessary.

Though I am loathe to recommend one insect repellent over another, most professional film people, guides, campers, and hikers seem to use Cutter Insect Repellent, as do I. I find it the most effective one to use, and I like it especially since it comes in liquid, stick, and spray form. The little plastic bottle fits snugly into one of my pockets or in my overnight bag, and it's not only effective against mosquitoes, but also against chiggers, ticks, flies, and those incredibly pesky little gnats that abound during the summer months down south.

Parenthetically, I might say a word about *anything* that comes in either liquid or spray form. It is difficult to carry an aerosol can of anything with you on a long, tedious trip. They cannot be packed in your luggage while flying, since they are illegal aboard the airlines and vulnerable to leakage. If the item comes in a glass bottle, transfer it to a plastic container, one that can be tightly sealed and locked, and either pack it in your flight bag or put it in an ordinary plastic bag and tie the top to prevent leakage. It's what I do with all my medicines, liquid cold-water detergents, and, of course, my insect repellent.

TROPICAL TRAVEL

- If the hotel in which you are staying provides a mosquito netting, there is generally a very good reason. I strongly suggest using it.

- Check the netting for any tears, rips, holes. Somehow, insects are quite ingenious in finding the one hole that exists in an otherwise impenetrable shield. The same holds true for the screens on the windows. If there is a tiny hole, the scotch tape you've brought with you (!) will seal it sufficiently to keep the insects outside. If you didn't bring scotch tape, try a band-aid.

Some years ago we were traveling through the Yucatan Peninsula in Mexico and our little jungle hotel did, indeed, have mosquito netting. It was the time before air conditioning (yes, Virginia, there was a time before air conditioning—television, too!), and the method used to cool the huts during the humid tropical nights was to wet down the thatched roof with a garden hose—the evaporating water would serve to take the temperature down somewhat. There were, indeed, window screens, but there were also a great many varieties of insects on the premises.

We checked the mosquito netting and I helped my wife into her bed, checking to see that there were no holes, tucking it in tightly around her and under the mattress, then turning to do the same to myself. I had no sooner gotten into my bed, my own netting firmly in place, when I heard the most horrendous scream come from my wife. For there *in the netting with her* was the biggest, greenest, ugliest, most menacing beetle I had ever seen. I had checked everything, it seems, except to see if she had any company with her *inside* the netting when she got into bed!

- In any tropical area, when you get up in the morning, shake your clothes out thoroughly and turn your shoes upside down, shaking them too. Clothing and shoes are the favorite nighttime sleeping places of scorpions.

- Make sure you shower with soap at least once a day, and even more if

215

the weather is unbearably hot. Then check your body carefully for crabs, ticks, and lice.

Of course, if you are one of those people who is allergic to insect stings, it would be wise to check with your doctor before setting off on your trip. This holds true as much for the United States as it does for the rest of the world, since yellow jackets, wasps, hornets, and even honey bees can be dangerous. One way to avoid being stung is to use some common-sense preventive measures.

• Don't use perfume, cologne, hair sprays, scented deodorants, or scented after-shave lotion, since they all have a tendency to attract insects. Unfortunately, some suntan lotions also attract insects, so you will have to decide whether you want to be tanned or stung!

• Don't walk around barefoot. I've seen many travelers who cover themselves completely with light clothing, and even wear hats, yet they walk around without shoes! Your feet are the most vulnerable part of you if you go barefoot—spiders, ticks, scorpions, mosquitoes just love your feet.

I once read an interesting item that said that more people get stung by bees around swimming pools than anywhere else. I suppose this is true at resort hotels and at many domestic vacation places, but the traveler into tropical areas stands more of a chance of being bitten by a greater variety of insects than the person who spends the bulk of time basking in the poolside sun. Which brings me to the more exquisite types of insects, the really menacing ones.

NEVER BECOME
FRIENDS WITH
THE ANOPHELES

Of course, if you are traveling to an unusual part of the globe, I assume—I genuinely hope—you will do your research and your probing beforehand about the types of insects and diseases that are prevalent in that part of the world. There are illnesses of the tropics with strange, exotic names—illnesses that are insect-borne, that strike at vacationers on the

Mediterranean coastline of beaches and resorts—and all of them are preventable by using a combination of insect repellent, proper clothing, and mosquito netting.

I will not go into an encyclopedic description of all of them, for your research will tell you whether or not that particular disease or insect is one to watch out for. Even diseases like filaria, spread by mosquitoes, forest flies, and the buffalo gnat, generally strike in the rural areas of undeveloped countries, rather than in the cities which most travelers tend to frequent. The same holds true for sandfly fever, dengue fever, and sleeping sickness (trypanosomiasis). All have varying effects, ranging from an unpleasant illness for the first two to the serious consequences of the bite of the tsetse fly for the latter disease. The average traveler will not be affected for the most part. If you are planning a trip out into the bush (as I did in Kenya), then make sure you check thoroughly about the prevalence of the disease in your area of travel.

Interestingly enough, not all of these insect-borne diseases occur in the wilds of the jungles. There is one that is quite prevalent in some resort areas of the Mediterranean coast, through Greece, Sicily, Portugal, Corsica, and even parts of the French Riviera. It goes by the name of kala-azar and it's caused by the bite of the infinitesimally small sandfly (too small, in fact, to be kept out by ordinary mosquito netting). The bite results in a high fever and some infection, and, here again, the use of insect repellent is a must.

There is one area, however, in which I would like to give a strong warning. The diseases mentioned above are really quite rare, though they do exist and they present a potential hazard to any traveler going off the beaten track. There is no doubt in the minds of international health officials that malaria, on the other hand, is once again on the increase. This is due to several factors. First of all, there are now some drug-resistant strains of malaria in various places of the world, but, more important, we have been finding that travelers are just *not being warned* about malaria before they go off on their trips.

HOW TO PREPARE WISELY

No one likes to set off on a journey with words of warning ringing in the ears. The tourist bureaus of the destination countries are loathe to mention the negative things about their countries, as are many travel agents who sell the package tours. All of this, combined with the ignorance of the traveler, the lack of preplanning and reading before leaving, and the common habit of "putting our heads in the sand," have given rise to a tremendous increase in the incidence of the disease.

But the frightening thing is that malaria is not only becoming more common in the undeveloped areas of the world, it is also becoming a threat in some of the temperate zones and modern cities as far north as New York! It is a frightening disease carried by the anopheles mosquito, and it's accompanied by headache, fever, chills, and sweating. But it can also cause anemia, heart or kidney failure, coma—and, in some instances, death. The tragic thing about it is that *it is almost entirely preventable* if you take the proper precautions before going into a malaria area and after arriving at your destination. The most obscene thing is that warnings are not given to the traveler by the experts who guide the choice of trips, of destinations, of resort hotels. If, on the other hand, the "experts" are also ignorant, then it is up to you to make sure you know everything there is to know about your trip before you depart.

Though I mentioned two sources of information earlier in the book (Chapter 3), this might be a good time to repeat them. Both give complete information about malaria areas. The first is the publication: *Health Information for International Travel* (HEW Publication No. CDC 79-8280), U.S. Public Health Service, Center for Disease Control, Atlanta, GA 30333. The second source of information is IAMAT (International Association for Medical Assistance to Travelers), and I will discuss this organization fully in the next chapter. They offer to members two excellent leaflets: *How to Protect Yourself Against Malaria* and *World Malaria Risk Chart*.

In addition, it's wise to keep these simple rules in mind:

• If you're going to an area where malaria is a threat, make sure you take your antimalarial pills before you start your trip, all during your trip, and after you return. (They are discussed in Chapter 3, and your family physician can help with a prescription for chloroquine, camaquin, or other medication.)

• When in the country, keep yourself covered and use insect repellent constantly. Sleep under mosquito netting and spray your room several times a day.

• The most dangerous time for the traveler is between dusk and dawn, when the mosquito is most rampant.

• Wear light-colored clothing at night, since the anopheles mosquito is most attracted to darker colors.

According to research done by medical investigators, about five million Americans and Canadians travel each year into areas that are high malaria risks. They range from Central America and parts of South America to Central Africa, Southeast Asia, and even into parts of the Caribbean. Meanwhile, back here at home, there is a most casual attitude about malaria, and the resurgence is a frightening sign that either the information is deliberately not being given to the departing traveler (try to find warnings about malaria in Caribbean travel brochures, for example) or there is an honest ignorance about the dangers of the disease.

More frightening, perhaps, is the fact that many of the hospitals and a great many doctors in North America cannot even recognize the symptoms of the disease! When you place this alongside the unfortunate fact that no one has a legal obligation to tell you that you are even traveling into an area of potential hazard, then you begin to understand why I feel so strongly about the responsibility being yours and mine. And I smile rather wistfully when I read a quote attributed to a government official in a country where six tourists recently contracted the disease: "Reports of malaria occurrences in (country) are highly exaggerated." Not, my good man, if you were one of the six!

And have I—I who take my spray, my mosquito netting, my repellent along with me, who take my malaria pills religiously—have I ever had a run-in with a hostile insect? Well, most of them are stories that every traveler has encountered, such as the one in the Yucatan that I wrote of earlier. But there was one incident that was not really preventable, I suppose, and it had a funny ending, as all good stories should.

We were working in the jungles of South America, on the Rio Magdalena in Colombia, and we followed all the precautions about food and water and mosquitoes. We were warned not to step off the jungle paths because of the "two step" (the mamba snake), called so because once you were bitten, you could take only two steps before succumbing to the bite (or so we were told). Along with that, we were there during the time of *La Violencia,* the revolution in which over 200,000 people were killed. So the prevalence of bandits was also a warning given to us while we worked. It was, to be sure, a lovely trip—once we were out of the country.

However, with all the precautions and the adventure, I came out feeling rather exhilarated and filled with stories waiting to be told. I arrived in Miami to visit my family and noticed that a large bump was beginning to form on my kneecap. Almost as I watched, it swelled and rose and filled with fluid until it resembled a miniature Mount Etna, about to erupt in lava and fire. I realized that I had probably been bitten by a spider on my last day in the jungle and I rushed to the telephone to ask my friends and family where I could locate

219

a doctor to treat it. I was certain that I was about to expire in an instant if I did not get it treated immediately.

There was only one problem. Miami doctors are obviously quite efficient when it comes to chronic disease, aches and pains, and sunburn. But no one seemed to know what to do about a spider bite. One doctor even suggested that I go to a dermatologist and he promised to call back when he had the name of one. I paced the room, the mountain growing larger on my knee, and the phone finally rang. I rushed to it, slid under the table, and, in doing so, the infection caught on the edge of the desk and erupted in one large, wet explosion! I looked down, horrified. The knee was slightly red, the spider bite was gone, and I was cured! Cured by the edge of a desk while answering the telephone. Put that in your medical books, if you like!

20

"AU SECOURS!" MEDICAL ASSISTANCE OVERSEAS

About the Occasional Medical Emergency and Some Organizations That Might Be of Help...

If you travel enough, there are bound to be times that you fall prey to the vicissitudes of the wayfarer. At times, it will be nothing more than a mild case of culture shock, and there is nothing that you or modern medicine will be able to do about it. While you wonder how it is possible that "anyone can live this way," just keep in mind that they have probably been doing it for as much as five thousand years and they're still around. Keep in mind, too, that as you are looking at them, they are also observing *you* and wondering how "anyone can look that way!" Of course, you don't need a doctor for culture shock.

The affects of the trip might also reflect themselves in malaise, Montezuma's Revenge, or a mild case of altitude sickness. Luckily, most of these symptoms are as fleeting as those of culture shock, and they will also be handled easily by you without the need for medical help.

There are times, however, when a difficult or even serious medical problem does occur and, depending upon the part of the world, there are various ways in which it can be handled. It won't be like a visit to your family doctor, but you might be very much surprised to find that some of these emergencies are handled even more efficiently, sympathetically, and effectively than the cases you bring to your own physician in your own city. Recently, there has been a spate of articles about medical emergencies in China, and each writer has been surprised and overwhelmed at the treatment and the low cost of the incidents. In some ways, the medical community of the United States and Canada is far behind the rest of the world in some areas of patient care, even given our sophisticated schooling and intensive training. Of course, in other parts of the world, be prepared for the most archaic of medical practices and get yourself back home as quickly as you possibly can, if the affliction will allow you to travel at all.

The carriers, both airlines and cruise ships, are well prepared for medical emergencies. The pilot of the aircraft is responsible for just how to handle them, and the decision to turn back, to go on to the final destination, or to make an emergency landing is one that has been made countless times. The one place that I feel completely safe about care and consideration should an illness occur is aboard one of the large jets. I have seen a pregnant woman go into labor aboard a plane in Asia, and I have seen the handling of a sudden death in Alaska, and both times I have been impressed with the calm, the efficiency, and the knowledge of the crew. And so, if I complain about airline food, I more than make amends in this chapter.

Ships are a slightly different problem, since they cannot quickly turn around or "land" at a strange port when an emergency occurs. All good cruise ships generally carry a doctor and nurse aboard, though freighter trips will not provide that service to the few passengers who travel with them. If you have a potential problem, check out the ship before you book the cruise. Ask about doctors, medical facilities, hospital accommodations should you need them, and emergency care while at sea.

I was curious about this area, since most of my travel is on jet planes. On my film cruises aboard Holland-America, I found their ships well equipped with doctors, nurses, hospital facilities, oxygen, EKG, and all other emergency needs. This seems to hold true for other modern cruise ships. The QE-2 gave me an idea of what an up-to-date ship now carries in order to service its passengers medically. Here are just a few examples:

• An examination room, a dispensary, and a laboratory equipped for bacteriological, biochemical, haematological, and blood transfusion work.

- An out-patient department in addition to a hospital of six wards, where all beds have dividing curtains. (I might also mention that each ward also has a TV set, for those of you who can't stand to miss one episode of your favorite sitcom.)

- An intensive-care unit, oxygen, nitrous oxide, operating theater, the latest in anaesthetic devices, dental surgery rooms, physiotherapy department, deep-heat-treatment equipment, and several X-ray units.

The list is incomplete, but I am amazed at the development of a system of medical care for ship passengers when I think back to my first trip overseas during World War II on a troop ship carrying 4,600 seasick soldiers and three barely trained doctors just out of medical school!

FINDING A DOCTOR OVERSEAS

One of the earliest travel tips given to me was the information that a medical emergency could best be handled by calling the American or Canadian consulate or embassy and asking the person on duty for the name and number of an English-speaking doctor. It worked then, and it still works as an emergency measure. The duty officer or the marine on post at the time will generally have an updated list on hand.

On a trip to Rome back in the early 1960s, my wife was stricken with her recurrent gastrointestinal spasms, something she picked up in Bangkok some years before. During a bad night, I telephoned the American embassy and got the number of an English-speaking physician, and—at three in the morning—he arrived at our hotel. He was dapper, suave, darkly handsome, sure of himself, charming, and efficient. His English was passable so that we could tell him that my wife was having severe stomach spasms. His bedside manner was impeccable, that of an Italian lover, and my wife fell madly in love with him at that instant. She does not even remember what he said or what he prescribed for the illness. She only remembers that she was treated by Marcello Mastroianni that night. I, in turn, tell her that she was delirious with fever and the only thing that I remember is the large bill he presented for his bedside manner. Possibly I was also a bit jealous, since I have been told that I resemble Keenan Wynn rather than Marcello Mastroianni!

But the advice about calling the consulate or the embassy still holds true

223

in most parts of the world, since someone is on duty 24 hours a day (except for those days when American embassies are being attacked by howling mobs).

If you are in an area where there is no consulate or embassy, your hotel will generally have a list of doctors on call, with specific information for nights and weekends. I prefer using the first source, or the list of doctors given to me by IAMAT, rather than the hotel, since I have no idea of the qualifications of the hotel doctor, nor do I know if he speaks English. How will I communicate my symptoms? Playing "charades" will only get you so far when you have to describe nausea, stomach cramps, and severe diarrhea!

There are other ways to find a doctor or a hospital if the emergency is severe and, for some reason, the hotel or consulate cannot help.

• Call the emergency room of a well-equipped hospital. In the larger cities, these are available on a 24-hour basis. Sometimes a large university or teaching hospital is also accessible. In fact, in dire emergencies such as a heart attack, it is wiser to get right to the hospital than to wait for the doctor to arrive at your hotel to make that decision.

• The international symbol for the location of a hospital is a sign carrying a white "H" on a blue background. I notice that we are also beginning to use this symbol on our highways right here at home.

• In rural areas or in cities that do not have modern medical facilities or readily available doctors, try to contact the local group representing any international organization. For example, many missionary groups have trained doctors with them right on staff. Failing that, the International Red Cross or the representative of a United Nations group might be able to help.

ORGANIZATIONS FOR MEDICAL ASSISTANCE

In the last few years, several organizations devoted to emergency medical care have been formed. Though everything I have mentioned already is still quite valid, I have found that belonging to one of the groups has solved many of my travel problems. They provide the best of up-to-date information about immunization, weather and dress, malaria conditions, and complete lists of English-speaking doctors around the world, from Algeria to Zimbabwe. Certainly, nothing is perfect in this world, and there have been instances of doctors not being available at the moment of need. But even the local telephone directory at home is is not completely up-to-date, and, overall, I found the medical groups to be the best possible source of overseas information when I had need of a doctor.

In fact, one night in Bogota, Colombia, I called a doctor quite late at night, after getting his name from the IAMAT booklet. (It was again my wife's Bangkok stomach that was acting up.) Within the hour he was there at our hotel, and he subsequently made three more visits. His fee was reasonable, and the big surprise was that he was a close friend of our family doctor back home, who had also practiced in Bogota right after World War II. The doctor has become a close personal friend and we have seen him on several trips to Colombia, again proving my theory of *piccolo mondo* ("small world"). Now, I will not guarantee that the use of any booklet containing the names of local doctors will result in such a charming ending, but I still smile when I think of the incident turning from one of a nighttime emergency into many lovely dinner parties over candlelight at his home.

International Association for Medical Assistance to Travelers (IAMAT). 350 Fifth Avenue, Suite 5620, New York, NY 10001. (The Canadian office for IAMAT is: 1238 St. Clair Avenue West, Toronto, Ontario M6E 1B9.) I have mentioned this organization several times in the book, mostly because I have belonged to it for some number of years. In addition, all the people in my traveling staff are members of IAMAT. The group provides competent medical treatment in over a hundred countries, with English-speaking doctors on call 24 hours a day. In addition, the fees are set for office visits and house calls, nights and weekends. Some of their literature has also been tremendously helpful to me before I set off on a trip: *Information on Health Hints, World Climate Charts* (that include information about water, food, milk, and clothing), *Malaria Risk Charts,* world immunization information, and—most important of all—the list of doctors recruited by IAMAT and who are on call around the world. There is no charge for the service, but they do request that you contribute whatever you can so that the work can continue.

Intermedic, Inc. 777 Third Avenue, New York, NY 10017. This organization works on very much the same principles as does IAMAT, and it comes just as highly recommended. They, too, offer a list of English-speaking doctors around the world. In some cases, in the smaller cities and towns, the very same doctor services both IAMAT and Intermedic, but for the most part, they each work with their own personal selections in every country. Fees for house calls, hotel calls, office visits, and weekend and night charges are also published in advance and given to their members. Intermedic subscribers, upon request, can also receive immunization information by visiting or calling the office. There is a small fee for membership, with special family and group rates available.

International SOS Assistance, Inc. 1420 Walnut Street, Philadelphia, PA 19102. This is a medical service group devoted, for the most part, to servicing the corporations that maintain large staffs overseas or have personnel who constantly travel around the world. They do work with individual travelers, but their concerns seem mostly to center on corporate accounts and group plans. They have medical service centers on five continents, with a reference list of English-speaking doctors on call, as well as emergency evacuation service with medically supervised repatriation, and emergency hospital funds, if needed. Their fees vary depending upon number of members, number of trips, and type of employment outside the United States. For the individual traveler, I would probably recommend IAMAT or Intermedic. However, if you are currently with a corporation that has many overseas offices or construction sites, you might want to look into SOS.

In an earlier chapter, I also recommended Medic Alert for those travelers who want to carry a tag giving medical information for emergencies. So that you don't have to go thumbing through the index again, here is their address: Medic Alert Foundation, P.O. Box 1009, Turlock, CA 95380. There is a small fee, and membership is deductible as a medical expense.

The other medical tag that I suggested was from Mediscope; it provides very much the same information, only it is enclosed in a magnifying capsule. Their address is: Mediscope Medical Information, Ltd., 243 East Shore Road, Manhasset, NY 11030.

If there are hypochondriacs among us, you will sadly take leave with me as I go on to other kinds of advice to make your trip "easy going." There is so much more to traveling wisely and well. It is time to move on, but before I tell you more stories about our hotels around the world, the ways to make life easier aboard the airline of your choice, and how to handle the languages of the civilized and uncivilized world, let me write these next few pages about an experience that I have been rather short with—travel in the United States.

SECOND INTERLUDE: THE AUTHOR THINKS OF HOME

———————— •◆• ————————

I went fishing off our island dock last night. The sky was overcast and the tide was just turning. The village was almost empty, for it is early spring as I write, and the weekend people disappear on Sunday nights and return the following Friday to open their houses to squeeze in every bit of pleasure for the short two days of isolation. The last boat to the mainland had long gone and I was alone as the fog rolled in, slowly obliterating the hazy image of the distant bridge and the lights on the shoreline almost seven miles away. It was quiet, so very still, except for the occasional raucous "screech" of a circling tern looking for an evening meal of inshore bait-fish. There were no other sounds, no other movement. There were, in fact, no fish biting either. But it didn't matter.

I looked around me, at the water, the boats riding at anchor, the now-dense fog covering the bay, the misty dock lights cutting a veiled path of light down to the dock, and I realized something that has struck me time and time again. If this were a foreign country, if I had discovered this in Europe or in South America, I would come home with the breathless tale of the little village at the side of the bay when the fog rolled in and covered the land. But this is home. This is where I live. I take it for granted too often. And yet, it is the equal, certainly, of anything I have ever felt or seen anywhere in the world.

I have gone through so many chapters of this book recalling the romance of foreign places, and I wonder if I have not been unfair to my own country. It is true that we destroy our history much too quickly by tearing down that which does not please us any longer. Either it is too old, too small, uneconomic, or just plain ordinary by today's soaring standards. Europe has learned to treasure its heritage. The temples of Asia are two thousand years old and they will be there two thousand years from now. Do you remember at all what stood in the middle of your own main avenue before they tore it down to make way for the fast-food outlet? Perhaps all this is what keeps us such a young and vibrant country. I do not know.

I complain about the food that I must put up with on the trips I take so often. I am upset that every motel in every town and every state looks very much the same as every other motel in every other state. If I do find charm, it is generally run down. If I do find grace, it is off the beaten track. And yet, as I stood on that quiet dock, I began to think of all the things in America that I have loved and cherished and spoken of and thought of time and time again during moments of meditation. I was very much surprised at the impressions that came back to me, and I would not have space in an entire book to list them for you.

I have complained about the sameness of our food, and its lack of imagination and care. And yet, what about the days spent in Maine, eating lobster on the piers for breakfast, lunch, and dinner! Lobster steamed in sea water in large drums. Where in the world can I find a taste that equals it, for every other lobster in every other part of the world is but a vague imitation of our own North Atlantic variety.

I have gone to markets all over the world, and any traveler on vacation also heads immediately to the Casbah or the Bazaar in Istanbul or the native market of fruits and vegetables set up under tar-paper roofing on every continent in the world. If I were a foreign visitor coming here, to these United States, how would I feel when I visited the Fulton Fish Market in New York at 3:00 A.M. to watch the catch come in, the shouting and the loud auctioneering by some of the most colorful people in the world? What about Pike's Market in Seattle, stretching for blocks under the long walkway near the waterfront? It is the equal of any I have seen anywhere. The French Quarter of New Orleans, the shrimp docks at Corpus Christi, the delicious Amish Market in Lancaster, Pennsylvania. Supposing I were a European being taken on a tour by an American friend—what would my reaction be and would I take it all for granted?

Supposing I had discovered Waxahachie, Texas, in some foreign country. It is the most incredible of gingerbread towns on the way from Dallas to Austin, and it's well worth the side trip to see it. I parked my car in the middle of the main town square to take a photograph of the brick-red courthouse, built after the Civil War and boasting the most charming statue of a small soldier in Confederacy grey on the lawn in front of the entrance. A woman stopped her car to watch and then spoke to me.

"Do you find that beautiful?" she asked.

I turned and smiled. "It's one of the most beautiful and interesting courthouses I've ever seen in this country. Yes, I do find it quite beautiful."

She thought for a moment, looked at the courthouse again, and said, "I suppose I've lived here so long that I don't see it anymore."

We produced a film some years back about the Lincoln Heritage Trail and our path wandered through Kentucky, Indiana, and Illinois, visiting the birthplace of Lincoln, his homes, the major historical sites. It was autumn and the festivals were taking place all over the area. I remember the whittlers sitting in front of the courthouse in Henderson, Kentucky, 30 or more older men just sitting and whittling. Nothing more. No real conversation. The concentration intense. Just whittling. I asked one of them what he was whittling and he answered, "Nothing'—just makin' little sticks out of big ones."

There are so many photographs, most of them in my head rather than on 35-mm slides. If I stop to think, they are all as exciting as any trip that I've taken to any place in the world. The small plane that flew through the Grand Canyon and then turned sideways to narrowly miss the Rainbow Bridge. A helicopter trip from Salt Lake City to Price, Utah, circling over snow-covered mountains on which elk ran wild, scattering before the whirling blades as we dipped down to take a closer look. The sunset over Lake Powell in Arizona and the one over the Slinden farm in Grove City, Minnesota, as we harvested corn late in the evening and I drove their truck to speed things up while my crew kept filming before the light disappeared for the day. To this day, I look at the film we produced there and, in the darkened screening room, when the image of the truck comes slowly out of the sunset and the combine pours its harvest into the back, I lean over and whisper to whomever will listen, "I was driving that truck, you know!"

It has been all of 35 years and there is more, much more. But it is not important here. It may well be the fodder for another book or I may just keep my stories to myself from now on. The thing that I most wanted to do was to write about what I felt was an omission of feeling, a love of travel that transcends the final destination. Many of the people I have met here have, for the most part, been as interesting as any I have come across in foreign countries, for there are both dull and exciting people everywhere in the world. And, possibly, just possibly, the communication here has been better than in most places because all of us speak approximately the same language. And yet, each section of this large country of ours offers a different heritage, a unique opportunity for discovery, a new world to which we can open ourselves. It's a beautiful place, this land of ours. Having said that, let us then move on to the business at hand.

HOW TO FLY DEFENSIVELY

About Airlines, Your Rights When Flying,
Some Problem Solving, Tips on Reservations,
Luggage, Smoking Rights, Delays, Overbooking,
Cancellations, and Complaints . . .

The newspaper clipping on the following page is yellow with age. I don't even know why I kept it, but I am, among other things, a squirrel, and I dug it out as a prime example of a case in which the passengers had very few rights aboard the airline. The old phrase "Go fight city hall" is quite meaningless when the city hall is in Nairobi! The story also has a humorous sidelight (now that we are so many years away from the incident).

There was no way to notify our contacts in Athens that the plane would be eight to ten hours late. I thought that once we arrived in Morocco I might be able to cable somehow, and so, on touchdown, I decided to leave the plane for the hour of refueling and send the cable (or at least get a soft drink). The Rabat airport was heavily guarded, ringed with howitzers and armed men. The king was taking no chances that any of his guests would be bothered. After the delegation had left the plane, I followed them and bounded down the steps in the hot sun, only to be met by a soldier carrying a mean-looking automatic weapon. He barred the stairs with his gun.

231

THE DAY WE WERE 'HIJACKED' BY E.A.A.

AS film-makers who travel in Africa a great deal we have a warm and genuine feeling for your part of the world. I must say, however, that you do try our patience at times.

On Saturday, June 10, our film crew was booked on EC 760 for Athens. We were told that the flight was non-stop and it was announced as such.

Once aboard the plane and in the air we learned that the Tanzanian delegation to the OAU had decided that the plane was to fly to Rabat and then to Athens. Rabat as you no doubt know, is almost eight hours from Nairobi. With no chance to change our plans and with important clients awaiting our flight in Athens (where, incidentally, they were given the wrong information about our arrival), we were taken to Rabat, not allowed off the plane, and then flown to Athens.

To say the least, it was illegal. However, I was interested in several other aspects.

On the very flight on which we were politically hijacked,

I read in the NATION that Mr. Kileo had made the following statement: "The sales promotion campaign of the airline is faulty because the corporation is full of foreigners who had an imperialistic attitude. Foreigners including pilots and engineers were here to destroy the corporation, not to serve the people."

Shakespeare would have said that Mr. Kileo is "full of sound and fury signifying nothing" for the only people who seemed to care about the passengers that day was the foreign crew.

It is unfortunate that fewer and fewer people will fly East African Airways. To further make my point I have sent copies of this letter to our travel agent and to others. I frankly do not expect anything to happen.

It is your prerogative to run your airline any way you see fit. It is our prerogative not to fly with you again.

Mel London,
Vice-president,
(Vision Associates,
New York).

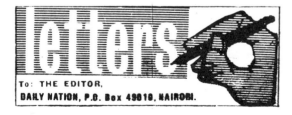

To: THE EDITOR,
DAILY NATION, P.O. Box 49010, NAIROBI.

"I think you had better go back, sir," he said rather politely but very firmly.

I put on my best air of haughtiness, taught to me by my British friends, and answered, "Look, young man. I didn't ask to be brought here, you know." Possibly it works with the British, but it cut no ice with the young soldier. He moved closer and became more menacing.

"I think you had better go back, sir." I began to think they were the only words he knew. I went back. We got to Athens ten hours late, to be met in a deserted airport at 2:00 A.M. by disinterested Customs people who finally let us through with our film equipment.

Of course, most airline confrontations do not involve political hijacking, armed resistance, and a letter to the *Daily Nation* in Nairobi. Nevertheless, not knowing your rights aboard the carriers can often mean a frustrating beginning to a planned vacation, a business trip gone awry, or a much-delayed arrival at your final destination.

AIRLINE RIGHTS

First of all, if you fly at all, I would suggest that you send for a remarkably concise and informative pamphlet issued by the Civil Aeronautics Board. It's called *Fly-Rights: A Guide to Air Travel in the U.S.,* and it's available at any CAB field office in the country. Or, you can get it by writing to the Civil Aeronautics Board, Washington, DC 20428.

International travel presents other problems. Though most major carriers are members of IATA (International Air Transport Association), complaints to the organization or letters to the main office of the carrier will get about as much response as a personal letter to the king of Morocco telling him how rude his soldier was to me. For international carriers, the best solution is to contact the U.S. office of that airline, since the competition is quite fierce on overseas routes and your complaint might get some sympathetic treatment. I will cover complaints later in this chapter.

RESERVATIONS AND TICKETING

The most misused word in the airline industry (as well as the hotel business) is "confirmed." You may have a confirmed reservation and you may have your ticket, but somehow you may get to the airport to find your flight

233

overbooked and your seat just not available. The most important thing that you can remember about travel is that you have to think things through—you must travel defensively, expecting that things might go wrong, anticipating what it is you have to do should they, indeed, go awry.

• Try to book your flight well in advance, and, if possible, have your ticket *before* you get to the airport. That way, you avoid the problem of crowds, the tension before departure, and, worst of all, "computer breakdown" so that your reservation is nowhere to be found. See that the flight is marked "OK" on your ticket.

• If you make your reservation by telephone directly with the airline, be sure that all information is repeated back to you (this has become standard practice with most carriers), that flight information is correct, and that dates are confirmed.

• Get to the airport early. You'd be surprised how this can avoid many of the problems of which I will speak later on. Check your luggage early, get your seat assignment early, and be on board promptly. If you are already in your seat and another passenger is "double-booked" for that seat, the airline must find another place for the later arrival.

Incidentally, should you lose your ticket, you are in for a long and complicated process. The ticket can be reissued, of course, but you must prove that you purchased it in the first place. It's a good idea to jot down the number

---

IMPORTANT

In the unusual event you arrive at an airline ticket counter with your ticket to find that the airline shows no reservation for you, DO NOT LEAVE THE COUNTER. Check your ticket. If the status box shows OK for the flight in question, the airline must accommodate you on that flight. If that is not possible, they must either find you a substitute flight, or pay you denied boarding compensation. If the problem persists, ask to speak to their supervisor or service manager. Remember . . . . if your ticket reads OK . . . . you are OK.

PORTS OF CALL   TRAVEL CONSULTANTS, INC.   To   *Saks Fifth Avenue*

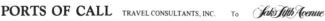

Notice to check for flight OK

of your ticket in a safe place—but it's a better idea not to lose it at all! Anyone who picks it up can use that flight or change it to another destination. Some refunds can take months, others are accomplished in hours. Should your ticket be used or cashed in, the airline may well refuse the refund.

LUGGAGE

In an earlier chapter, I suggested that you label your luggage with the return address of your office rather than your home. I might also suggest that if you use curbside check-in, you wait until the skycap brings the luggage to the moving belt or inside the terminal. We are very firm on this because our film equipment is worth so much.

• When the tags are put on your bag, make certain that all other tags from previous flights are off the luggage, and that the new tags do, indeed, list your final destination. Look carefully at your stubs.

On the other end, if your luggage does not arrive, you must contact the supervisor before you leave the terminal building. The airlines will insure each bag for $750, but they usually demand receipts or sales slips when you make your claim, if they feel that you may be inflating the value of your loss. The most difficult part of it, though, is that the airlines seem to take forever to pay—sometimes it can stretch into months.

• If you are on a stopover and your luggage does not arrive, you can ask the airlines to pay for the essentials needed to tide you over until it (hopefully) does. But, as in every case that follows, *you must ask* and you must ask strongly. The airlines have an unfortunate habit of doing nothing until it is demanded by the passenger.

Sometimes the bag is merely delayed, of course, and it will arrive on a later flight. Make sure you stay in touch with them and demand that the bag be delivered to your hotel. There is no need for you to return to the airport to pick it up.

• If your bag is damaged on the trip, the airline will pay for repair. This can also be a big pain, since you will have to get to your hotel, unpack, and then take the bag to the shop recommended by the airline. There is, unfortunately, no way out. If the bag is damaged when you check in, or if

235

the handle is broken, a "damage" tag will be attached to your luggage to show the handlers at the other end that, for once, it is not their fault.

SMOKING OR NONSMOKING

I remember rushing to the airline counter on my way to somewhere. The agent took my ticket without greeting me, asked for my preference of a seat, and then, upon hearing my answer, solemnly announced: "I'm sorry, sir. We don't have any more nonsmoking seats available." In an equally imperious voice I told him that he would therefore have to make the *next* row of seats a nonsmoking section. He grumbled at this interloper who knew the rules—but he complied.

Again, this is a prime example of the airline never telling you your rights. You must know them in advance. On all American carriers today, they must offer you a nonsmoking seat if you so request it. If the "no smoking" seats are completely filled, then the next row must, on request, be made a part of that section. On many international carriers, however, the old rules still apply and you will no doubt find people puffing away all over the plane, day or night. Grin and bear it. One day it will change, just as it did on domestic carriers.

DELAYED FLIGHTS

There is nothing that you or the airlines can or will do about flights that are delayed due to bad weather, fog, mechanical difficulties, or late arrival of aircraft. There are days when the entire country is blanketed in fog or ice or snow or hurricanes and every plane at every airport in the country is delayed somehow. Some years ago, over the Christmas holidays, just such a thing happened—for four days! The entire country was covered in fog and ice from coast to coast, and if you speak to the airline employees who were working that memorable weekend, you will see their faces turn pale at the thought of the hundreds of thousands of passengers who were stranded at their airports!

• If your flight is to be delayed for several hours, the airline will generally pay for a call to your final destination. Again, you may have to ask.

236

- If the flight is delayed overnight, the airline will pay for a hotel room, assuming that the airport is not your own home town.

- Vouchers are generally issued for meals at the airport restaurant if the delay takes you through breakfast, lunch, or dinner. In addition, they will also provide transportation to a hotel if it is necessary to stay the night.

The delay may be inconvenient or frustrating, and I have heard much grumbling at airports when they were closed due to fog. But an Act of God is not reimbursable. However, when I feel that the delay is due to a mechanical problem at some distant airport, while every other flight seems to be going out on time, I try to rebook if I can. Airline employees sometimes do not know the reason for the delay, or they just will not impart the information when you inquire. After all, a lost passenger represents lost revenue. There are times I have felt that this principle is more important to them than having a satisfied passenger.

IF YOUR FLIGHT IS OVERBOOKED

The airlines do have a problem, of that there is no doubt. Some passengers book and then don't show up. Others unfairly book three and four flights under different names to be sure they get out of a city after a business appointment no matter when the meeting ends. By law, the airline is allowed to overbook—to sell more seats than the plane will hold. For the most part, the system works, believe it or not. I don't know how many times I have been "stand-by" on a completely sold-out flight, not only to finally be boarded but to see empty seats around me. However, you ask, suppose everyone shows up? Aha! That, too, has happened, and someone just isn't going to be aboard when the flight leaves the terminal gate.

- The best solution for the overbooking problem is early arrival at the airport. When a flight is overbooked, it is the last arrivals who suffer the consequences.

A new system has been put into effect with regard to the overbooking and "bumping" problem. The airlines are now required to ask for volunteers to give up their seats in return for compensation and a seat on a later flight. Though my army career taught me never to volunteer for anything, I find that many others are more than willing to give up their places when the request is made.

• The airline can decide just how much to offer the passengers who so volunteer. All the employees of the carrier are given guidelines, but the amount is finally negotiated between the agent and the passenger. I watched one bidding session go from $50 up to $125 before a passenger would give up his seat.

NOTE: To show how quickly "new systems" become old systems, however, the rules were changed again just as this book was going to press. The Civil Aeronautics Board has made a ruling that an airline (domestic or foreign) can compensate a passenger by offering a free flight instead of a cash payment. Under the new policy, the airline has the option of offering the bumped traveler a voucher for a free flight, or a check, or cash, in addition to honoring the ticket that the passenger was unable to use. The moral of the story is that things happen too quickly in the volatile airline field to keep up with them. Make sure you ask—make sure you demand to know your rights if you are bumped. No one will ever volunteer the information to you!

If you do have the time to spare and if you are willing to become a voluntary "bumpee," be sure to ask the airline some questions before you give up your seat:

• If the delay is to be a long one, will the airline provide meals, a hotel, phone calls, taxi fares?

• In fact, just how long a delay are they talking about in the first place? When does that next flight leave and will they guarantee a seat on it?

• If the airline hedges on that last question, offers to place you on stand-by because the next flight is full—keep your seat. You're better off where you are.

And so, the next question is: "Suppose no one wants to get off?" The airline will then resort to an involuntary bumping, generally one of the last passengers to arrive. The new rulings, however, require that the airline compensate the passenger for the inconvenience, and it's usually based upon the length of the delay and the amount of your ticket.

- If you are bumped involuntarily, the airline must pay you the cost of your ticket plus a minimum of $37.50 up to a $200 maximum.

- The airline must arrange a flight to your destination within two hours of your original booking (four hours on international flights) or the compensation doubles.

You will still keep your original ticket and you can either turn it in for a refund or you can use it at a later date to make another trip. Here again, you must know your rights, because the chances are that the agent will not let you know how much they have to pay you and just what it is you can expect from them.

There are also several exceptions to the bumping rules. Your reservations must be confirmed in order to qualify; you cannot be wait-listed or on stand-by. If you arrive at the boarding gate just as the plane is about to taxi off the ramp, you probably will have no claim of being bumped. (Remember the homily about always arriving early?) If the airline must substitute a smaller plane on the route for some reason—for example, replacing a 727 with a DC-9—they will not have to pay. (Get there early!)

IF YOUR FLIGHT IS CANCELLED

Essentially, the rules here are the same as those for delayed flights. The airline is responsible for getting you on another flight or, failing that, to put you up at a hotel outside your own home city, feed you, and generally see that you get out of that airport at the first possible moment. This can be a rather trying experience in some parts of the world or during the worst times of holiday travel.

There are rare instances, though, where there is some minimal compensation for the delay. Several times over the past years, I have had flights cancelled overseas and the airline has placed me in the first-class section at no additional charge, since they were the only seats available on the next flight. Do keep in mind, too, that the airline has absolutely no obligation to compensate you should you miss an important business meeting, or if your vacation is delayed for a day or two while the hotel room at your destination goes unoccupied (though paid for).

THE ART OF COMPLAINING

There is no doubt that dealing with the public in a service business can be frustrating at times. Not every passenger is a paragon of good sense and politeness, not every passenger takes the time to understand what the problems of the airlines might be. Take any Christmas rush through a major city like Chicago or New York or Los Angeles or Atlanta. Add to the normal increase in traffic the unforeseen delays due to weather, overbooking, late arrival of aircraft—then put yourself in the place of the agent behind the desk who has been working 12 straight hours trying to get everyone to a final destination in time for Christmas dinner.

Nevertheless, under normal circumstances the passenger does have a right to complain—and complain strongly—about some of the treatment given at airports, aboard the planes themselves, and at the other end of the line. Being irate doesn't help. Jumping up and down at the ticket counter in front of the harried agent is another way to be promptly ignored, your demands unmet. The very best way to handle any complaint situation with the airlines is to ask for the top person on duty. The passenger service representative has more clout than the agent, is generally a middle-line executive or supervisor, and is used to handling and solving passenger complaints. Generally, most travel problems are solved right there on the spot, and the passenger goes off a bit disgruntled, but on the way nevertheless.

If you have not solved the problem at the airport, then it is time to write a letter to the airline, making certain that you have all the facts written down: time and date, flight number, names of airline personnel with whom you've dealt, and any out-of-pocket expenses you may have incurred (try to have receipts, if possible).

Get the name of the highest airline executive you can—even the president or chairman of the board. It all goes along with the theory that you go as far up to the top as you possibly can. Write to that individual *by name,* not by title alone. A simple phone call to the airline office will get the information for you. To be sure, you may not receive a personal letter from him. And then again, you may. (I have gotten many return letters from airline presidents once they learned that most of our company travels over 150,000 air miles a year. A customer is still a customer!) In any case, if it has his name on it, there's a good chance that it will have been read in his office and passed down to another executive.

• Make your letter succinct and businesslike. Don't just take his time by griping about what lousy service the carrier gives.

• Give details, enclose copies of documents, stubs, and so forth.

• Be reasonable and state what it is you would like them to do about the problem.

This step will solve still more of the common problems encountered with the airlines. You might indicate that you are sending a carbon copy of the letter to your travel agent so that the information is also conveyed to someone who will be booking many airline flights for passengers for years to come.

Still no satisfaction. You have received a lovely form letter telling you that they are terribly sorry and that they "will take it up in training." There are other methods to follow through with, though—and each one puts still more pressure on the airline. Through it all, however, remember that you don't want to acquire the reputation of being a crank. Keep your tone throughout as businesslike, straightforward reportage.

I remember taking a trip to Manila via Tokyo on one of the worst, most-crowded, worst-serviced flights I've ever been on in my life. I do write complimentary letters at times, incidentally, but the letter to the airline president on this occasion was one of the most ironic and vitriolic I'd ever composed. The flight, to put it bluntly, was a nightmare for a variety of reasons. Sure enough, about two weeks later I received a personal letter from the airline president, apologizing profusely for the inconvenience and enclosing a check with which I was, according to his request, to take my wife out to dinner, compliments of the carrier. I did accept his apology and I was charmed by the gesture, even though the check was not enough to buy dinner for *two* in expensive New York. The thought was there, however, and that's all that counted at the time.

WHAT YOU CAN DO ABOUT IT

We will assume, for argument, that your complaint is more serious and you still do not receive adequate apologies or compensation from the airline. It is time to move further.

241

• You can write to your state's attorney-general's office, your state department of consumer protection, the local Better Business Bureau, or the local newspapers, TV, and radio hotlines. Airlines do not like that kind of publicity.

• Here are some other letter addresses—and this time, make certain you send a carbon copy to the president of the airline in question, just so the airline knows you are going further: Consumer Information Office, Interstate Commerce Commission, Washington, DC 20423; Bureau of Consumer Protection, Civil Aeronautics Board, Washington, DC 20428; American Society of Travel Agents, Consumer Affairs Department, 711 Fifth Avenue, New York, NY 10022.

• If the complaint that you have is about a safety-related incident anywhere in the airline system or aboard an aircraft, write to: Community and Consumer Liaison Division, APA-100, Federal Aviation Administration, 800 Independence Avenue, S.W., Washington, DC 20591.

• A copy of all letters should be sent to your travel agent.

As a final resort, you may have to go to the small claims court in your area, but I frankly have heard very few stories where the complaints have led that far. Usually, somewhere along the line, you will get satisfaction. It is much easier for the airlines to settle a complaint with a dissatisfied customer, especially if the passenger is in the right—which all of us are all the time, are we not?

As we move on and we reach our destinations, you will find now that many of the same problems that plague the airline passenger also manage to follow us right into our hotels around the world.

22

NO ROOM
AT THE INN

Naturally, About Hotels, Motels, Reservations,
Some Tips on Security Away from Home . . .

I am firmly convinced that every hotel and motel in every part of the world has what must be called the "American Room." I first became aware of it many years ago while traveling in Europe. We'd get to the lovely villa overlooking a magnificent lake (complete with fishermen out in their full-sailed skiffs), drive up the winding path to the front door, be greeted like visiting royalty by the staff, and then be shown to a room at the back of the hotel, overlooking the morning garbage collection and a brick wall built to hide the nearby open-pit strip mining. If the hotel was on the Grand Canal in Venice, they always found some way to present us with a room that looked down on a back alley, regardless of what the reservation letter stated. If the establishment was, in turn, on the bustling main thoroughfare of an exciting metropolis, the room was located on the inside air shaft and one had to climb over the bed to get to the closet on the other side of the cubicle.

At first I thought that it was my hostile face that created all of this, making it necessary for me to go storming back to the front desk in order to have the room changed (which it most always was), thus starting my trip on a very sour note. I realized after a number of years, however, that it was not *me*

243

they were picking on, it was my *nationality*. I was being given the American Room—I obviously didn't know any better and I obviously would not complain. Well, a lot of years and a lot of room changing and a lot of miles have passed since then, and though the practice is still as common as ever, there are ways to circumvent it, the most effective one being a simple ploy learned from my European friends:

- Don't go directly to your room along with your luggage. Leave the bags well guarded down at the desk, possibly with the bell captain, and then ask to see your room before you take your key and accept their first choice. I have actually had desk clerks change their minds as soon as I made the request, muttering something about "a mistake" and handing the bellman another key for a better room.

- If you don't like the room they show you, ask them for another. They may well tell you that there is nothing else available. There usually is something else available and firmness can pay off.

I remember arriving in Brussels late one night for a ten-day business stay. At that time, I usually booked an older, charming hotel at the edge of the city, because the rooms were large and spacious and the beds were quite comfortable. That night, however, I was led to a room that could well have been the classic American Room. It was about seven feet by eight feet, with a large bed filling most of it; I could get to the bathroom only by crawling across the bed, and the bathroom door could not close because it had no room to swing. I looked in horror and anticipated spending ten days in that prison cell. (Of course, the window also faced an air shaft.)

I promptly marched down to the desk, muttering obscenities and thinking of a famous joke that travelers like to tell:

"I'm sorry, sir, but we have nothing else."

"Well," the frustrated businessman answers, "What if the queen were coming tonight?"

"Oh, sir, I'm sure that we'd find something for her!"

"Well, the queen is not coming. Give me *her* room!"

I arrived at the desk determined not to use that old saw, but just as determined that I would have my room changed, no matter what. The conversation began as expected.

"I'm sorry, sir, but we have nothing else."

He explained that I had checked in late, that there was a horse show in town, that they were, indeed, fully booked except for my little room. Nothing that I said could sway him. I began to think that he was telling the truth (or that he was the master of the desk clerk lie). I decided to try one more tack, to appeal to his pride.

"This hotel is part of the Ritz chain, is it not? The Ritz in Madrid is also one of your hotels?" He nodded and I continued, "Well, I find it hard to believe that the Ritz chain would give such a room to an old customer!"

Somehow it worked. He looked at me for a moment, then turned his back to look at the key board. In mock surprise, he exclaimed, "Aha, here's one that I had forgotten." The room, to say the least, was superb, a small suite for exactly the same price as the cardboard box into which I had been put.

It is interesting to note that the American Room does not only exist in Europe and the other foreign continents. The same thing takes place right here in the United States and Canada. They may not call it the American Room, though I do, but it always overlooks an air shaft, the same smelly garbage dump, or some other malodorous pit. Room clerks generally are instructed to fill those rooms last, but I guess they feel that if they fill them *first,* they won't have to worry about having them left over at the end of the day.

There are, of course, some ways to avoid the American Room in advance, though I still strongly suggest that you not take your luggage to your room until you've checked it out—here or overseas.

- Reservations are a must. Try to make them far enough in advance so that you have time to receive a letter of confirmation from the hotel or motel.

When an establishment is overbooked, it's an easy matter for the desk clerk to tell you, "I'm sorry, sir (or madam), but I don't have any record of your reservation." I don't know how many times in the past 35 years I have had to whip out the manager's personal letter welcoming me to his hotel in order to convince the desk clerk that I did, indeed, belong there.

- In the United States, particularly, the assistant manager on duty in the morning generally selects reservations with special requests as the first order of the day—river view, away from the highway, king-size bed, small suite, and so on. You have a better chance of staying away from the American Room when a special request is made at the time you reserve your room.

There are many ways to find out just what the hotel or motel offers. The Michelin guide for French hotels and restaurants is one of the best in the world for that particular area of Europe. Almost all other guidebooks also recommend and rate hotels. In the United States, the American Automobile Association (AAA) guides and the Mobil guides are the best on the market, and each gives a fairly complete description of the accommodations and the amenities. In addition, your travel agent has all the materials at hand to give you further information, including the *Official Hotel and Resort Guide* that describes and rates over 25,000 hotels, motels, and resorts throughout the world.

The governments of the countries to which you will be traveling may also rate their hotels and have the information available on request. Unfortunately, ratings are very vague and inaccurate in some parts of the world, and "first class" may mean one thing in one country and another thing somewhere else. Even the ratings of "de-luxe," "first class," "second class" (or "tourist"), and "third class" may not mean much, depending upon your destination. Make sure you state the kind of room you want, whether you want a private bath or are willing to share one (if, in fact, the hotel has any private bathrooms at all), and ask what meals are included in the rate. Some hotels require, during the height of the season, that you take at least breakfast and one additional meal with them. If you like to wander and find the local restaurants and taste of the native cooking, as I do, this can be a very severe handicap. Make sure you find out the check-in and check-out times, too.

RESERVATIONS

• Most hotels will only hold a reservation until 6:00 P.M. unless other arrangements are made in advance, or unless you telephone from the road to tell them that you are delayed and will be checking in late.

And, therein lies another travel problem. If you are foolish enough to travel without reservations, be prepared to be turned away from hotel after hotel (or motel) when you hit a town where a convention is taking place or it is the height of the tourist season near Yellowstone Park. I know many people who love the serendipity of not knowing where they're going to spend the night, but I also know of many who have spent the night in their car, along with the dog and the kids. If you do travel that haphazardly, then you already know that you must stop early in the day, while the motel signs still carry the Vacancy sign.

For those of us who do travel with reservations, we still are not problem-free. There are times when the room is not there, even though you have booked it in advance, you carry a confirming letter clutched in your hot little hands, and you have been traveling all day looking forward to a hot bath and a good dinner. Hotels, like airlines, overbook to account for no-shows. Sometimes too many people show up and the computers have a headache. No room at the inn for you, the late arrival. Smugly, hotel owners and their association tell us about prepays and guarantees. I would like to spend some time writing about this, for it is, without doubt, one of my pet peeves. Finally, I have a chance to air my unhappiness about it.

"GUARANTEES"

One way to "guarantee" a room is to prepay the first night. This is especially important at vacation resorts (and, in fact, some demand it), overseas hotels where you may be delayed in arriving, and even for convention trips. Most of the time it works. The hotel is already paid for the night and they will hold your room for you until you arrive, no matter how late it is. Even here, you must understand, the system is not foolproof. We once arrived in Hawaii after being delayed in Seattle by fog for almost six hours and the luxury hotel in Waikiki had given our rooms away! We were late, after all, and it was treated as being our fault. The hotel was filled, the room clerk turned his back and walked away, and I called to him rather sharply. In this particular case I had an answer that I could only use that one time.

"You don't understand, young man. We are the film crew who have come here to do a motion picture about your hotel! Part of our story is the service you offer."

His face paled and somehow four ocean-front rooms were located within the next five minutes. We had, indeed, been hired by the hotel chain to do a public relations film on that particular resort.

The other side of that coin is the "guaranteed" reservation. Most business people use it, but there are occasional times when it just does not work. When the reservation is made, the room is guaranteed. In other words, you can arrive at any time during that night and the room will be kept for you. Should you not show up, you must pay for the room either by the credit card you've registered with them or by check. But, just imagine a lonely desk clerk in a dimly lit hotel lobby at midnight. You have not shown up as yet. The clerk is confronted by another lonely traveler who needs a place to sleep, so he gives your room away, certain that you will never be there. He is thus able to get your guaranteed payment *plus* the revenue from the other traveler.

Your plane arrives at 2:00 A.M. and you make your way wearily to the hotel, only to find that your guarantee has meant nothing. At this point, all the hotel and motel owners and their associations throw their hands up in horror. Give away a guarantee? Never! Well, hardly ever! They retort that they, in turn, must find you an equal accommodation somewhere in town. But if you have ever seen the "equal" accommodations they find for you, as I have, you would be just as upset as I am at the problem. One motel in California found us "equal" accommodations at the local house of prostitution (or a facsimile thereof).

HOW TO COMPLAIN

What can you do about it? Well, you can write letters, as I have, and they will do you just as much good as my letters have. Which, to put it bluntly, means absolutely nothing. The motel and hotel associations are not government-regulated, as are the airlines, and you'll probably never be back again anyhow. In essence, they have entered into a contract with you that *you* must fulfill, but for which *they* have no legal obligation if they do not abide by their agreement to hold that room for you. It is, in essence, a "one-way" contract, and I am just waiting for the day when some large business group brings a legal class-action suit for all of us who have had to go through late-night arguments in deserted lobbies to convince the clerk that we were going to take off our clothes and sleep on the lobby couch unless a room was found. For the most part, something does get done. But we are not always so lucky.

The best defense against the habit is to do as I suggested earlier: Get a confirmed and written guarantee—get the name of the clerk who takes your reservation on the telephone and then jot it down—then reconfirm a short time before you are to arrive, and firmly state that you will be arriving late and that you want the room held. It only lowers the odds. It is not "guaranteed" to work.

Hotel and motel stories abound. Business travelers and tourists regale one another with tales of lost reservations, corridor adventures, and funny incidents. I remember traveling to Corpus Christi on a job about a year ago and it was the first time that my client (a woman) and I were to be together for any length of time. We enjoyed the flight down there, even though the connection out of Dallas was about two hours late and we thus arrived at our motel about midnight. The sleepy desk clerk looked vainly for the reservations, but somehow (!) they were not to be found. All he could come up with was one double room. Leering across the desk, he whispered, "I only have one room. Wouldn't you two like to share it?" I answered in about five short, succinct words and he somehow located the other, missing room reservation.

SOME THINGS TO BRING WITH YOU

Earlier in the book, I suggested some things that might make your hotel stay more comfortable, and I would like to mention some of them briefly again—with a few additional tips.

• Most hotel rooms were never designed for applying make-up. I would suggest that you take a portable, lighted make-up mirror with you to enhance the dim light of the hotel lamp.

• Don't forget a small transformer if the area uses 220 volts rather than the normal 110 of the United States and Canada. That goes for adaptor plugs, too.

• Take along a night light to plug into the wall socket for that nocturnal trip to the bathroom.

• Have a small flashlight with you if you don't take the night light.

• I have a friend who actually buys bulbs right at her destination so that she can exchange the dim, low-wattage ones with a brighter variety. Not a bad idea for reading at night.

And, if you're going overseas, keep in mind that making international telephone calls can be terribly expensive. Though the basic rate is fairly reasonable for three-minute calls, the hotel will frequently add on its own service charge, bringing the cost up to double or triple the listed rate. Ask what the cost is before you make the call, or send a night letter cable to tell everyone you've arrived safely.

Some years ago the Bell System, in conjunction with the major hotel chains, instituted a system called Teleplan, designed to hold down the costs of international telephone calls. Each member of the group agreed to charge their guests only a reasonable surcharge for the call. If Teleplan is in effect in a hotel, it will be so listed. If it is not, be careful, and don't forget to ask about the cost.

The other method of making an overseas call is to have your party or business associate call *you* from the United States at a given time. Frankly, unless I am in a larger European city, I try not to make overseas calls, since placing them and getting through may take hours of waiting in my room for the connection to be made. London and Paris are easy, but Quito and Bogota are nearly impossible.

AND ABOUT SECURITY

Security is an area of potential paranoia, or a subject that can be handled—again—with some good, common sense. There is no doubt that you and your belongings are more vulnerable when you travel than when you stay at home at a backyard barbecue. Nevertheless, most of us have been traveling for years over hundreds of thousands of miles with only an occasional mishap, and that usually due to our own ignorance or stupidity.

I remember the days before credit cards, when we had to take thousands of dollars in traveler's checks with us in order to pay the bills for a film crew of four people over a period of two to three months. I once made the mistake of leaving my checks in my room (thinking they were hidden). While I was out, some clever hotel thief took two checks *from the middle of the book,* thinking that I would never miss them and, even if I did, I would be far, far away from that city when I did find out. As it turned out, I counted the checks each night and also double-checked the numbers, so the loss was made good the next day at a branch of the bank that had issued the checks. But it was a good lesson, and I carried those traveler's checks with me each and every day from that point on—even though they made my pockets bulge as if I were carrying billiard balls.

The first thing I strongly recommend is that you take out a travel "floater" with your insurance agent before you leave on a trip. They're quite reasonable in cost and they'll give you peace of mind while you're traveling. I carry one that covers me and my personal belongings, and I buy it on a yearly basis. All of our film equipment is, of course, also covered by insurance for our work overseas.

- Don't carry large amounts of cash with you. Also, when you purchase traveler's checks, treat them exactly as you would your cash. Make note of the numbers and put this list in a safe pocket, away from the checks themselves.

- Make note of your passport number in case it is lost or stolen. It will help get you a new one with a minimal amount of trouble.

- If you're carrying jewelry or other small valuables, use the hotel safe

250

deposit box. But first make sure that you find out what the hotel's limit of liability is.

In some countries I go so far as to wear a money belt for the cash that I am carrying with me. These places are generally where I know that I will be working or traveling through crowded city streets or in some of the worst areas of the country. Actually, my cash is probably safer in the smaller villages than it is in the middle of the urban metropolises.

• Carry your wallet in an unfamiliar place if you are going to mingle with crowds. The theory behind this is that you will feel the bulge if it is in a pocket where you normally would not carry it. In that way, you will always know it's there.

• You will probably have some credit cards with you. Make certain you also have a listing of those numbers in case the cards are stolen. Before you leave home, you would do well to empty your wallet of all the credit cards you won't need while you're on your trip. Your local bank cards, department store cards, and service station cards will not do you much good overseas.

Your hotel room should also be considered as a potential target for thieves, and there are a few things that you can do to make it more difficult for them.

• Lock the door securely before you go to sleep. If there is a chain or bolt, use it.

• When you check into the room, take note of the fire emergency exit near you. I have been in three hotel fires in my travel life and I find that I now automatically note the exit staircase, even if I am on the fifty-third floor of a skyscraper hotel.

• If there are sliding doors that have access to a balcony, patio, or pool, make sure they are also locked.

• Be careful with your key, and make sure you don't advertise your room number in public places.

• Don't invite strangers to your room, no matter how charming they may seem on that first meeting at the café or museum. Have your first rendezvous in a public room.

You are inevitably warned not to leave valuables in your room when you go out. Of course, this caution is fairly easy to follow for jewelry and smaller objects, which can be left in the safe deposit box or taken with you. But it becomes awkward if you follow the rule implicitly and you have to take your large camera and accessories out to dinner with you.

Here is where the paranoia comes into play. You don't want to ruin your trip by constantly worrying every time you leave the hotel. If your larger valuables and your clothing are covered by insurance, if you are carrying your traveler's checks and cash with you, you will be taking as many precautions as are practical under the circumstances. However, here are some other suggestions:

- Put the Do Not Disturb sign on the door before you go out. No intruder will really know if someone is inside and he or she probably won't take the chance of entering.

- Double-lock the door. You will notice that many locks in foreign countries can be turned twice to double-bolt them.

- The sign reading Maid: Make Up Room is a dead giveaway that no one is inside.

- Hiding valuables in the drawers, under clothing, in a locked suitcase will not deter a thief. The suitcase can be kicked or pried open easily, and leaving it unlocked may well show a potential thief that there's nothing in there worth taking anyway.

- If you go out of your room for even an instant, if only to go down the hall to get soda or ice—lock your door. It takes just a moment for a thief to take your valuables.

I think that the most vulnerable time for any traveler is when the day of departure arrives. We pack our suitcases, leave them on the beds while we go down for breakfast, and then come back upstairs to gather our things and leave the hotel. If anything is taken during that time, it will probably not be discovered until we are thousands of miles away, or even back home. That is the time that I put the Do Not Disturb sign on the door and take my valuables with me.

252

THE "IDIOT CHECK"

Since my crew and I move in and out of hotel and motel rooms so much, there is a tendency to become overconfident, to consider ourselves easy travelers who are at home most anywhere. And it is that overconfidence that creates some of the problems. We therefore have instituted what we call the "Idiot Check" and it is performed religiously whenever we leave any hotel to continue on our journey. The Idiot Check is nothing more than making sure that we have taken everything with us—film equipment, personal belongings, valuables, even our directions to the next destination.

After we've packed, we check the drawers again, we look at the bathroom shelf, behind the bathroom door (ah, how many bathrobes have been left behind in that hidden place!), under the beds (for shoes), and in the closets for anything that might have fallen on the floor during our stay. In spite of all this, I once had to turn around when I was one hour out of San Francisco to drive back to the hotel because I knew instinctively that I had left all my shirts lying in the bureau drawer (even after the Idiot Check)! I put the incident down to a creeping case of senility and I have since been victim of the barbs of my crew, who now snidely ask as we leave: "Are you sure you took your shirts?" Boldly, I answer "Yes!" But underneath it all, I do wonder. Did I, indeed, take my shirts from the drawer?

23

"MY GOD! IT'S NOT ALL GREEN!"

*Various and Sundry Things About Money,
How to Exchange It, and How to Tip*

———————————◆•◆————————————

Before we discuss why all foreign money looks like the payments made in a Monopoly game, stop for a moment to consider the dilemma of the overseas visitor to the United States. *All* of *our* paper money is green, and all of it is the same size! Think about that for a moment—$1, $5, $1,000 bills totally the same, albeit with different pictures and numbers on the front. It's no wonder that our foreign friends complain that they're always peeling off the wrong denomination to pay a taxi driver or give a tip. Frankly, it makes more sense to have different colors and even different sizes for currency, as most every other country in the world does. You may not be used to it when you first arrive overseas, but you'll soon find it practical and simple.

Another interesting psychological thing begins to happen to Americans traveling overseas. Since the money *looks* strange and since it seems to have no intrinsic value, there is a tendency to spend it just like the Monopoly money I teased about. Never fear, it *is* real money, as you will soon find out when you try to total up how much the trip cost you and you realize that you've overspent by double your estimate.

PREPARATION
BEFORE YOU LEAVE

Learn the values *before* you arrive. Learn to convert dollars to the local currency and back again, so that you can determine in an instant whether that pair of shoes in the shop window really is as reasonable as it seems to be. There are currency guidebooks and tipping charts available, but be warned that this volatile world sees exchange rates vary from day to day, frequently at an awesome pace. The exchange rate given to you in the guidebooks will be an estimate, and only that. Generally, you will see the daily rate posted in your hotel or in a nearby bank or currency exchange office.

When you arrive at a foreign airport, unless you are with a group tour that is taking care of all tipping, transportation, and check-in at a hotel, you'll need to have some foreign currency to get you through the first few hours. Certainly, there are bank branches or government exchange offices at many airports, but the lines are generally long and your luggage is just coming off the carousel. The last thing you want to do is to stand there and wait your turn. In addition, many of these offices are only open during the daylight hours and your plane has just arrived at midnight.

- Before you leave, get some of the foreign currency, even a small amount—about $20 to $50 worth. This will get you through the airport, allow enough to tip properly, and then get you into the hotel. If you are to arrive on a weekend, get a larger amount, since banks will probably be closed on Sunday.

There are two places that can accommodate you in the exchange of currency right here in the United States. Both are reliable and both have helpful pamphlets available for their customers. Deak-Perera is the largest foreign exchange company, and there are offices all over the world. You may contact them at their World Headquarters: Deak & Company, Deak-Perera Building, 29 Broadway, New York, NY 10006. Their small booklet, *Foreign Money Converter,* gives current information on exchange rates, currency regulations, time conversions, clothing sizes, and even international road signs.

Manfra, Tordella & Brookes, Inc., located at One World Trade Center, Suite 3331, New York, NY 10048, came up with a most ingenious addition

255

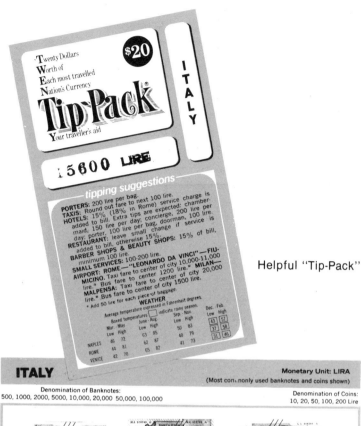

Helpful "Tip-Pack"

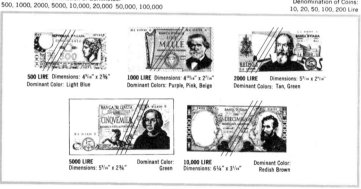

ITALY

Monetary Unit: LIRA
(Most commonly used banknotes and coins shown)

Denomination of Banknotes:
500, 1000, 2000, 5000, 10,000 20,000 50,000, 100,000

Denomination of Coins:
10, 20, 50, 100, 200 Lire

500 LIRE Dimensions: 4⁵/₁₆" x 2⅜"
Dominant Color: Light Blue

1000 LIRE Dimensions: 4¹³/₁₆" x 2⁷/₁₆"
Dominant Colors: Purple, Pink, Beige

2000 LIRE Dimensions: 5⁵/₁₆" x 2⁷/₁₆"
Dominant Colors: Tan, Green

5000 LIRE
Dimensions: 5⁵/₁₆" x 2¾"
Dominant Color: Green

10,000 LIRE Dimensions: 6¼" x 3¹/₁₆"
Dominant Color: Redish Brown

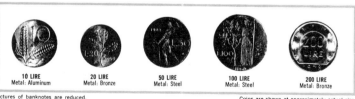

10 LIRE
Metal: Aluminum

20 LIRE
Metal: Bronze

50 LIRE
Metal: Steel

100 LIRE
Metal: Steel

200 LIRE
Metal: Bronze

Pictures of banknotes are reduced.

Coins are shown at approximately actual size.

Foreign currency identification

to the comfort and ease of the traveler—their "Tip-Pack." Each little packet contains a given amount of currency for the country, and carries tipping suggestions right on the front as well as reduced-size photos of the bills and coins; currency conversion tables are on the back.

CHANGING MONEY OVERSEAS

When you get to your destination, there are some other currency tips that you might think about.

• Always change your money at banks, American Express offices, Thomas Cook offices, or government-run exchange shops. The rates at your hotel are almost always a few percentage points below that of the banks. The reason is that the hotels must protect themselves against the daily fluctuation. Another reason is that I think the hotels are convinced that the traveler doesn't know any different anyhow.

I remember arriving in Rome just recently and I had not, as usual, followed my own advice. It was late Saturday night when we got there, and, coming from Yugoslavia, I had not had time to get some Italian lire for the couple of days until the banks opened. I figured it wouldn't make much difference, only a few percentage points—until I got to the hotel cashier's desk! The legal rate was nearly 900 lire to the dollar. The hotel was still giving *620 lire,* the rate of over five years ago. When I showed my annoyance, the clerk just shrugged. Take it or leave it? I took it and muttered under my breath.

• If you're really stuck, you can also exchange traveler's checks or U.S. dollars right in some shops or restaurants, but, again, the rate will be much lower than that of the banks or exchange offices.

Of course, there are exceptions. I gave a celebration dinner for some friends in a small town in Turkey. I checked ahead to see if the restaurant would take a credit card and they said they would, so we booked the table. The owner was a friend of friends, so the evening promised to be a festive one.

We dined well, drank the local wine, had a merry time, and I asked for the check, converted it into dollars mentally, and gave them my charge card. The waiter looked blankly at me. They did not accept charge cards. Well, then, where was the owner who was the friend of my friend? He had gone home.

257

There must have been some misunderstanding. They had never seen an American Express card nor had they ever seen Diners Club International. I whipped out my traveler's checks. I think they had never seen those either. They would not accept them. Somehow, I could see myself washing Turkish dishes for two centuries or so. The language problem seemed insurmountable and we were at an impasse—when the owner returned. Yes, there had been a mistake. They really did accept credit cards, but they didn't like to take them. Cash was better—no percentage to pay. He apologized. Again I muttered under my breath.

THE BLACK MARKET

• Never, but never, exchange your money on the black market. If you're approached by corner money-changers or people who hang around your hotel, turn them down. There are many good reasons. Most important, the black market is always illegal and the security police may well be posing as the friendly neighborhood banker.

In some countries, you are given an official receipt each time you exchange money legally. Save them all. Don't throw them away. You are liable to find that when you arrive at the airport on your way to your next destination, you will be asked for those slips with the official seal stamped neatly in the corner. No paper, no exchange back to U.S. dollars. Most of the time, this is a ruling that will not be told to you until it's too late. You can see why that's also another reason to stay away from the black market.

CREDIT CARDS

• If you use credit cards, remember that the rate of exchange of the day you used it is *not* the rate which the company will charge you. The exchange rate on the day the charge is processed will be the one passed on to you, and, in a volatile money market, you may be in for a big surprise. Use your card with care.

UPON RETURNING

When you complete your trip, you may have some foreign currency left over. It's difficult to compute just how much you'll need to get out of your hotel, tip the porters, take a taxi to the airport, and get your luggage to the counter. Some airports have banks available on departure, some countries may require that you show your on-going ticket (showing departure date) or the exchange slip you got when you first converted your money, and some will not allow their currency out of the country at all. If you have foreign currency left over, you may then be able to exchange it at the next point of arrival or, at worst, you can hold it until you get home. The two companies I listed earlier will be happy to buy it back from you in the United States.

After all these years, I play a little game with foreign currency. The trick is to see how *little* I can have left when I finally board the aircraft on my way out. This requires mental calculations that would frighten Einstein. But there is a method to accomplishing the feat. When I leave home, I take about $50 in U.S. currency in my wallet, all in small bills. I never touch it during the trip for any expense; I keep it for my departure magic. If I am short by only a few dollars, rather than exchange a large traveler's check and be left with too much foreign money, I quietly slip out the extra dollar or two to make up the difference in what I owe. However:

- Don't forget to ask in advance whether or not there is an airport departure tax when you embark. Some countries charge from three to ten dollars or more, and many will not take U.S. currency. The problem with these expenses is that you generally are not warned about them, and you only discover the small booth with the large sign when your hand luggage is going through the security check and you have had your passport stamped with an Exit visa.

HOW MUCH TO TIP

There is a general feeling around the world, well-founded to be sure, that Americans tip too much. Either that, or there is a feeling that Americans don't know how to tip at all. It is one area in travel where we tend to feel very vulnerable. We are, after all, strangers in the country, but we would like to look knowledgeable, act as sophisticated people-of-the-world, leave with echoes of "thank-you" ringing in our ears, and feeling that we have done exactly the right thing. Too often we do not. If we undertip, the staff grumbles. If we overtip, the staff does not really respect us very much. How to tip?

There is much that you can learn while still back home. The tipping

259

guides, the travel books, the Tip-Pack mentioned earlier are all a good beginning. Start by reading them carefully.

- Some countries add a service charge to the bills at restaurants and hotels. Sometimes it is quite sufficient. In other places, an additional tip is expected.

There are times that the service charge is added to a restaurant bill and you are expected only to round out the amount by adding a few coins. And there are also many hotels where the service charge is added to the bill, but the staff never sees a penny of it.

- If I have a friend or a contact in the country, I always ask the tipping procedure from the first moment that I enter the country. If you are not lucky enough to know someone there, ask your concierge or hotel desk clerk what the customs are.

- There is another simple procedure for your first time in a strange restaurant, and I have used it often. Look around you and find a table where someone is just paying the bill. Watch what is done: Is there small change left over in the plate when the bill is paid? Does the host, on the other hand, scoop up all the remaining change and pocket it, leaving nothing on the plate? It's fun to do and it gives you a feeling of how the natives handle their tipping.

Of course, the above suggestion is only valid if the people at the other table are not Americans and they, in turn, are watching *you* to see how you tip!

But above all, don't be intimidated. Once you have decided what you are going to tip, do it boldly, do it well, and smile!

ENGLISH (NOT) SPOKEN HERE

On Foreign Tongues

There was this mother cat who was walking along the road with her four kittens following behind her. All of a sudden there was this vicious bulldog right in front of her. She gathers her wits and shouts "woof! woof!" The dog is so frightened that he runs away. The mother cat then looks triumphantly at her kittens and says, "Do you see the advantage of knowing another language?"

J. I. Rodale
How to Choose a Marriage Partner

Foreign languages are one of the great frustrations of my life. I have studied French in school (and failed the course three times), have taken private lessons in Spanish (and just barely get along), and have worked and lived in Italy over a period of years, only to hear my close friends ask, "Mel, tell me, why do you speak Italian so well in restaurants and so badly everywhere else?" I suppose I just do not have the ear for it. Berlitz would not even accept me, judging me a hopeless case.

I look with envy upon friends of mine who speak 5 languages fluently.

261

My secretary in Italy wrote and spoke 6 tongues. An Indian friend of mine was master of 14 languages, including some of the most difficult in the world, like Japanese. Oh, I try. I do try. And I sit there in blind frustration while I think I am pronouncing the name of some restaurant dish quite correctly and the waiter looks at me in a total blank, not understanding at all. My language facility is so bad that I am beginning to doubt my English!

Of course, I minimize my insufficiencies by telling myself that there are some countries where people will not believe that an American can speak their language, even if he can. Japan is one such example, and most Japanese will just not accept the fact that *any* Westerner can speak their difficult tongue. A friend of mine, fluent in the language, worked in Japan for almost 15 years and he constantly ran into the problem.

One day, on a busy Tokyo street, he stopped to ask a gesticulating traffic policeman for directions. He asked the question, of course, in Japanese. The policeman kept directing traffic while perched high above the street on his wooden box. Again my friend asked the way to his destination. Again he was ignored. Finally, a bit frustrated, he shouted the Japanese phrases again. The policeman looked down, annoyed, and shouted back, "No spik Engrish!"

There are also times, I tell myself, when it is really wiser *not* to speak the language. Some years back, while working in Portugal under Salazar, the police would run nighttime roadblock auto checks—without warning, always with menace. Suddenly, I would come around a corner on my way home late at night only to see the wavering flashlights and the uniforms come up to the car demanding that I stop. My Portugese friends would say nothing, while I would grin, and in English greet them with "Good evening" while I handed over my papers for inspection. One of the police would mutter "stranger" in Portugese and I would be waved on. They never smiled back, but it didn't matter.

There's no doubt that if you speak the language of the country to which you're traveling, you will have a distinct cultural advantage. But if you were to work in 60 or 70 countries all the time, there's no way to be fluent in every language. (That is another thing I keep telling myself, to soothe my frustration over failing French.)

THE PHRASE BOOKS

The travel phrase books vary in effectiveness. Some are much too complex, and you would never have the time to find the sentence you need at the time you want it. I remember the first phrase book I ever used was given to me in the U.S. army during World War II, and it's totally valueless now. After all, who wants to know the French phrase for: "Which way to the 258th Signal Light Construction Company?" Instead of a phrase book, I prefer to carry a pocket-size language dictionary.

I find that there are also problems with the picture books that try to teach the language to incompetents like me. By the time I locate the picture, the situation has changed. I have found the following tips useful, and, if you are a total language cipher as I am, you might try them for yourself.

MENU TRANSLATORS

• The trick to survival is to know how to order in restaurants. (That is why I spoke Italian so well when in a *trattoria* and so badly outside!) Get yourself a good menu translator. There are several on the market and you can tear out the section that deals with the language you'll need on your trip.

When you buy the translator, make sure that most of it is devoted to giving you the name of the dish in the foreign language followed by the English translation, rather than the other way around. It stands to reason that you'll be translating menus that are written in the native tongue and you'll want to know if you are eating horse or pig, sheep's eyes or goat's tongue.

The Japanese have solved the problem, as they have solved many other problems in their own ingenious way. All over Japan, in front of every small restaurant and cafe, you will find a display of the foods they serve, sculpted in plastic, a pictorial menu that lets you take the waiter or waitress outside and point to the dish of your choice. On one trip, I was so fascinated by the ingenuity and the workmanship of these plastic replicas that I finally located a workshop outside Kyoto and bought a sample. On my table (among my souvenirs) is the most life-like plastic reproduction of a large banana split, complete with toppings and fruit!

HOW I SURVIVE AND COMMUNICATE

• Take your language book and transfer the important phrases onto three-by-five-inch index cards. It is easier to get to a card to find a quick phrase than it is to thumb through an entire book. And, as you pick up more phrases, you can add them daily.

263

My own cards are divided into:

- Everyday phrases, such as greetings.

- Directions (right, left, straight ahead), and how to *ask* directions.

- Numbers from 1 through 1,000.

- Simple, everyday phrases, such as "How much?", "Do you speak English?", "Fill the tank."

- Restaurant phrases, of course.

And then, the best trick that I have learned to make me sound like a native for 20 seconds is to learn how to say "I would like" and "He would like" and so on down the line until I can communicate the phrase for everyone in the group. The reason is simple. If I know how to say "I would like" then I don't have to know how to conjugate all the verbs, do I? Since I am a believer that every verb and every phrase in every language is an irregular verb, this saves me a great amount of trouble. Here's how it works:

- To the phrase "I would like . . ." I merely have to add the infinitive form of the verb, without conjugating it at all. "I would like . . . to eat . . . to drink . . . to visit . . . to drive . . . to go . . ." and a hundred other verbs that give me a head start in the new language. It also makes me sound a bit more intelligent when I order from a menu and I can say "I would like . . . the beef, the fish, the soup" rather than sounding like the stumbler that I actually am. Here are some examples in Spanish and French to show you what I mean:

SPANISH		FRENCH	
I would like:	*Me gustaria . . .*	I would like:	*Je voudrais . . .*
to eat:	*comer*	to eat:	*manger*
to take:	*tomar*	to take:	*prendre*
to send:	*mandar*	to send:	*envoyer*
a towel:	*una toalla*	a towel:	*une serviette*
breakfast:	*desayuno*	breakfast:	*petit déjeuner*
lunch:	*almuerzo*	lunch:	*déjeuner*
dinner:	*cena*	dinner:	*dîner*

The system also works with the opening phrase "Do you have . . ." or "Have you . . ." (*Tiene usted* . . . or *Avez-vous* . . .). For example, "Do you have . . . a menu . . . a car . . . change for 50 francs . . . a pillow . . . my laundry . . . a map . . ." And on, and on, and on.

As I said, I do try. I order breakfast in the language if I can, and I try the telephone calls in the language, and I do try to ask for my room key in their tongue. There is also an interesting thing that I've noticed around the world. Unlike Americans, people almost everywhere speak a second language (and sometimes a third). In Yugoslavia, for example, you may be able to get along in German. The same holds true for Asia, where English and French are spoken quite consistently. I have not yet learned how to say "I would like . . ." in Thai or Urdu, however.

Another thing that I try to do is to read the newspapers in the country I'm visiting. If the typeface is recognizable, you'd be surprised how much of the language you can pick up. Watch the television set while you're dressing for dinner; though you'll probably be seeing American reruns dubbed into Swahili, it's a good way to become familiar with the cadence of the language and its sounds, something that the newspaper cannot give you. Actually, I find that when I watch the politicians of many countries giving their speeches, I can understand more of the language than at any other time. The reason, obviously, is that all politicians speak to us as if we are three year olds, and if a child can understand it, why can't I?

ELECTRONIC LANGUAGE COMPUTERS

Recently, there has been some publicity about a new electronic pocket computer system that lets you translate a language by merely punching in your English words and getting the foreign response in a steady flow across a small screen (or vice versa). Frankly, I would not recommend them to any traveler. They are expensive; they are very slow; and they are limited in what they can do. By the time you punch in your phrase and then see it translated, it is very much like the picture books for language—the situation has long since passed. The final disappointment came when I was checking out these computers after the newspapers carried so many stories and advertisements about them. I thought that my salvation was finally here. The three-time French failure would only have to purchase a pocket-sized instrument that would make me fluent overnight. I was, at that time, frequently working in South America, so

I sped over to the New York department store that had placed the ads and approached a bright-looking clerk to ask about the Spanish language.

Around us, potential customers were busily playing with the little black boxes. The clerk chose the one with the Spanish cartridge. "Great little gadget," he enthused. He showed me phrases like "Where is the toilet?" and "How much does it cost?" and various other tidbits. It seemed awfully slow to me. He pooh-poohed the thought. Once I got used to it, he said, the speed would astound me. I took it from him to play with it myself and I punched in the word *peligro*. It slowly crawled its electronic answer: "Not on file." I looked at the clerk and he looked a bit perplexed.

"It means 'Danger'," I told him softly.

"Uh huh—well, maybe you spelled it wrong."

For a moment, I doubted my observation of the spelling of all the "danger" signs I'd seen around South America, warning me of various and sundry catastrophes. We threw the switch to English-Spanish and I punched in "danger," and it just as slowly said to me: "Not on file." I returned the computer to the young man and went home to locate my little three-by-five file cards.

And so, I will never be a linguist. I will never achieve the ultimate, as my friend Brian Bryce did in Asia by learning Cantonese in only nine years! I, along with all of you, will do the very best I can. If I find that I can't make myself understood, if I can't communicate no matter how hard I try, I will merely follow the advice of my good British friend, who advises: "When I don't understand the language, I merely speak English more loudly!"

25

"TODAY IS THE DAY WE WASH OUR CLOTHES"

The Ever-Present Problem of Laundry and Dry Cleaning — If You Dare!

I had never thought of a laundromat as a social gathering place—at least, not outside my own home city. We were in the darkest, most isolated part of Maine, one autumn night. The little village was, for the most part, deserted, the summer residents having gone home almost six weeks earlier. There was no local movie house, so we drove 72 miles to try to catch *Dr. Zhivago,* and arrived too late (7:30 P.M.) for the last show. It had started more than an hour before! So we drove back to our village and looked for where "the action is." The supermarket was just closing its doors and the local restaurant had long since shut for the night. The only bright spot in town seemed to come from a store a bit down the main street, so we headed over there and walked in.

It was the local laundromat, and it was filled to capacity with gossipy, chattering natives of the area. We had stumbled into the only social public gathering in town, and we spent a delightful hour chatting and exchanging stories and answering questions like: "How can anyone live in such a crowded place like New York?"—countered with "How can anyone live in so isolated a place like Maine?"

Laundry is an easy problem to solve when you're traveling in the United States or Canada. If you do your own, the little stores can be social oases as well as the magical solution to turning those bags of dirty clothing into clean, fresh, shining garments. I saw one laundromat that had a pool table in the back to keep the customers occupied during the "wash cycle." At another one, in Utah, the entire film crew left their bags of laundry with the motherly woman who ran the place, to pick it up fresh and folded later that day when we had finished our work.

The hotels and motels in the United States and Canada do make life easier for those of us who travel so much. Normally, if you turn your bag in early in the morning, the laundry will be back by evening, neatly pressed, with only an occasional sock or shirt lost to the gods. Overall, I have had good luck, though one member of my film crew is constantly losing a pair of trousers whenever he turns in his laundry. He has lost pants, to date, in North Carolina, Washington, Illinois, New York, and California. Needless to say, he always has at least one spare pair of trousers squirreled away in his suitcase.

"LAUNDRY DAYS"

To anticipate our clothing needs for a trip, we generally figure our "laundry days" as well as our travel days. This is a good idea for anyone taking a trip. If you know that you can send your laundry to a hotel on a given day, you can then anticipate just what clothing you'll need (counting lost trousers, of course). We exclude Saturdays and Sundays in the count. If there are no substantial laundry days in the trip, then we resort to packing a huge amount of clothing or going to the local laundromat at night. Incidentally, whether you are traveling or you have a home washer-dryer, there's an excellent booklet available that covers washing and drying tips as well as how to remove the most common stains on bleachable and nonbleachable fabrics. Since I am a slob, among other things, I have my own personal copy. It's called *Laundry Procedures* and it's available from the Home Economics Department, Maytag Company, Newton, IA 50208.

You'll notice that I have avoided mentioning dry cleaning, for I am terribly suspicious of the process anywhere outside the major cities and I do not trust the hotel services. Somehow I think they are chosen on the same basis as U.S. government contracts—the lowest bidder wins. I don't think I've sent out dry cleaning in a hotel or motel in 15 years, ever since a pleated skirt of my wife's came back without pleats and a pair of my trousers came back totally pleated! I have seen the "seer" taken out of the "seersucker," zippers mangled, and the classic case of a pair of white slacks that was returned with the complete burn mark of a hot iron right on the seat of the pants.

Another problem is that the insurance payments for damage are generally so low that they will not pay for replacement of the garment. Use your judgment on using the dry cleaning services. Possibly you have more faith than I do.

THE LAUNDRY JUNGLE OVERSEAS

In doing laundry overseas, there are no rules. It is every traveler for himself (or herself). The stories are hysterically funny, many of the laundry lists almost totally undecipherable, the service mostly unreliable, the methods completely "foreign" (no pun intended) to any American or Canadian. After a trip through the continents, your clothing begins to take on its own distinctive coloration, mostly due to the laundries you've run across.

- In India, they embroider your room number right onto the garment, each and every one. You carry a constant souvenir of your room numbers along with you when you leave the country. Only recently, I came across a pair of shorts with "923" neatly stitched onto the seam. I cannot, for the life of me, remember where I had room 923.

- In Australia, they steamed my room number on with a tag, and now, years later, each time I try to remove the tag, the fabric comes with it.

- The Europeans use thread of all colors to identify your particular laundry.

In many parts of the world, every shirt comes back without buttons. Or with broken buttons. When you realize that your hotel laundry is being done by women who are smashing the fabric on the rocks down by the river to get them clean, you begin to understand why you need a lifetime supply of extra buttons in your travel kit.

But the most hysterical part of it all for the traveler is the deciphering of the laundry lists that are left in your hotel room. It is late at night, you are sorting the laundry that has collected over the past few weeks, and you study

269

PALACE HOTEL

BRUXELLES
—

No 8566

BLANCHISSAGE - LAUNDRY

Chambre N° .... *Bruxelles le* .... 198 .

Madame ....

Pièces	DAMES	LADIES		Frs
	Chemise de jour simple ..	Chemise	15	
	Chem. de jour ouvragée ..	Fancy chemise	20	
	Chem. de jour tricot soie .	Silk knitted chemise ...	25	
	Chemise de jour soie ..	Silk chemise	30	
	Chemise de nuit simple	Night dress	20	
	Chemise de nuit ouvragée	Fancy night dress	25	
	Chem. de nuit tricot soie	Silk knitted night dress ..	25	
	Chemise de nuit soie ...	Silk dress	40	
	Chemise pantalon simple	Stepin	15	
	Chemise pantalon ouvragée	Fancy stepin	20	
	Chemise pantal. tricot soie	Silk knitted stepin	20	
	Chemise pantalon soie ..	Silk stepin	20	
	Combinaison simple	Combinations	20	
	Combinaison ouvragée ..	Fancy combinations	20	
	Combinaison tricot soie ..	Silk knitted combinations	25	
	Combinaison soie	Silk combinations	35	
	Pantalon simple	Plain drawers	15	
	Pantalon ouvragé	Fancy drawers	20	
	Pantalon tricot soie ...	Silk knitted drawers	20	
	Pantalon soie	Silk drawers	25	
	Jupon simple	Petticoats		
	Jupe ouvragée ou plissée .	Silk petticoats		
	Jupe soie simple	Fancy petticoats		
	Cache-corset simple	Camisole	15	
	Cache-corset soie	Silk camisole		
	Soutien-gorge	Bust bodice	12	
	Matinée simple	Dressing jacket	25	
	Matinée ouvragée	Fancy dressing jacket ..	30	
	Col	Collar	12	
	Col. ouvragé	Fancy collar		
	Bas	Stockings	10	
	Bas soie artif. ou naturelle	Artif. or naturel Silk stock.	15	
	Mouchoir	Handkerchief	5	
	Mouchoir soie ou pochette	Silk handkerchief	7	
	Blouse lingerie	Blouse	40	
	Blouse soie	Silk blouse	50	
	Blouse soie plissée	Fancy Silk blouse		
	Robe	Dress		
	Robe ouvragée	Fancy dress		
	Costume toile	Linen costumes		
	Jupe toile	Linen skirt		
	Tablier sans manches ...	Aprons		
	Tablier avec manches .	Pinafore		
	Peignoir de bain	Bath robe	30	
	Gants	Gloves		
	Serviette hygiénique	Sanitary towels		
	Pyjama	Pyjamas	30	
	Pyjama soie	Silk pyjamas	50	
			Total Frs	

Le montant de cette note sera porté sur la note de l'hôtel. La Direction
informe MM. les voyageurs qu'une seule blanchisseuse est admise à l'hôtel.

PALACE HOTEL
BRUXELLES
—

Chambre N° ....

No 8566

NOTE DE BLANCHISSAGE

COMPTABILITÉ

Total Fr. ▓▓▓▓▓▓▓▓▓▓▓

Bruxelles, le .... 196 .

the list by the light of a much-too-dim bulb. The Kyoto list asks you how many *tabi* you are sending in. You finally translate *pantalone* as "trousers" in Lima, but it takes some time to realize that the Italian *reggipetto* are "bust bodices," whatever they may be. What about "camisknickers" in Britain? How many "strips" are going to be laundered in Venice? I walk to the closet to check to see whether my raincoat is a "rain-coat-of wool," a "normal-rain-coat," a "sport-rain-coat," or a "two-sides-rain-coat" in Marbella, Spain. I finally decide not to send it in at all, since I think it is wiser to let it remain filthy until I return home and can give it to my own neighborhood dry cleaner.

- Before you turn in laundry to a hotel overseas, make sure you determine just when it will be returned. If they don't do one-day service, you may not have time to pack it in time for your departure.

Most laundry all over the world will be returned to you slightly damp. We have developed the theory, as yet unproven, that the only reason is that the laundry really wants to prove that they washed your clothing. If it's still damp when it gets back to your room, it must have touched water somewhere. You will also notice that all restaurant napkins in Italy are damp, probably for the same reason.

DOING YOUR OWN

Overall, except in the top de-luxe and first-class hotels, the laundry service is so unreliable in so many ways that many travelers much prefer to do their own wash. In spite of the fact that I work a full day on most trips, and though I send some work shirts out to the hotel laundry no matter where I am (meaning that I, too, am usually without buttons), much of my own washing is done right at the hotel. My kit includes the paraphernalia that I suggested much, much earlier in the book, and it's the easiest way out:

- A strong, thin line of nylon or other twine to hang across the bathtub.

- A plastic bottle of cold-water detergent, or the little individual packets that are now available.

Opposite, laundry list from the Palace Hotel in Brussels, Belgium

271

- A spot remover.

- Plastic clothespins.

Some people also like to take a traveling iron, which may be rather heavy in the long run—and you then also need a transformer, though you may already have brought one for your hair dryer. If you wear natural fabrics, as I do, you might just want to let them remain wrinkled for your everyday wear rather than ironing your laundry each evening. If you wear the man-made fabrics, just let them drip dry on the line or on the shower rack over the tub.

I also came across an ingenious idea that I have not yet tried. (It is reprinted here with permission, courtesy *Glamour*, copyright © 1976 by The Conde Nast Publications, Inc.) Barbara Gillam, Travel Editor of *Glamour* magazine, suggests that, having no iron with you and being unwilling to have the hotel press the pleats out of your pleated skirt, you remove the lampshade on the table lamp in your hotel room, dust the bulb, turn on the light until it gets hot, and then run the wrinkled garment over the top of the bulb. She claims it will take out some of the worst wrinkles very quickly.

I must try it the next time my *tabis* are crushed!

26

AMONG MY SOUVENIRS

*About Shopping, Bargains and Not-Such-Bargains,
and About U.S. Customs . . .*

I am not known among my acquaintances as the most erudite and selective of shoppers. I have left it to my wife and friends to choose the lovely things that decorate our home—the French fabrics, the tailgate of the colorful turn-of-the-century Sicilian wagon that hangs above the fireplace, the exquisite handmade Spanish masks to cover the faces of the picadors' horses during the bullfight, the clever Chinese tea warmer near the fireplace, the tiny emerald ring in a setting of gold that closely resembles the most delicate of sea shells.

SHOPPING FOR "BARGAINS"

I, in turn, am like the little boy let loose in the toy shop. My own collection is an eclectic jumble of insignificant and mostly unfunctional trivia, each one carried back from a trip as a prized trophy of my journey. You may sneer at my collection, but they were, each of the items, chosen personally by me and they are as precious to me as another traveler's ten-carat diamond, discovered in an Antwerp jewelry shop to be brought home and placed immediately in the family vault. Possibly, I even like my souvenirs more since they are so incredibly valueless that no thief would ever think of stopping on his way out to place them hurriedly in his sack of loot.

In addition to my little 40-cent Vietnamese vegetable peeler, I can look around me and see:

• My glorious collection of hats, from Brazil, the Middle East, Africa, the Amish country, Hong Kong, and Australia.

• A penny-whistle bought on a street corner in Johannesburg.

• My Masai spear that hangs on the wall next to my Colombian machete (made in Germany), and my billy club picked up after a riot in Asia.

• Finger cymbals from the Middle East, a sesame seed toaster from Japan, and a straw coconut-milk press from the Caribbean.

• A papier-mâché, three-horned bull mask painted in brilliant colors and found in San Francisco de Yare in Venezuela. It was made by a deaf sculptor to be used for the Festival of Corpus Christi, and I carried it with me in a shopping bag through seven Latin American countries over a period of a month, never letting it out of my sight. I carried it, in fact, straight through U.S. Customs in Miami, the three horns still sticking out of the top of the bag.

There is one souvenir which I no longer have, unfortunately. It was one of those marvelous "bargains" that I discovered in Nanyuki, Kenya, and which I bought for only 75 cents. It was a leather shirt and I adored it, until I got it home and my wife discovered it was filled with rat turds and vermin, so under pain of death or worse, I did get rid of it.

Shopping is a personal thing. Each of us goes abroad with an idea of just what it is we would like to bring home with us. No author can give complete advice on the subject, since not only are tastes different, but each country offers a different range of bargains and best buys—and even these change from time to time. The best that I can do is to give you some generally sound advice based upon my own experience, that of my wife, and on the travel stories of film people who keep coming back to tell me "how things have changed in Hong Kong" (which they have).

REGISTERING CAMERAS

• Before you depart for overseas, make sure you register your cameras, tape recorders, and calculators with U.S. Customs at the airport of departure. Most of these are now foreign-made, and it will save you time and trouble to have the evidence on hand when you return to this country.

Also, before you go, try to make up a mental list of all the things that you'd like to buy overseas—especially the high-priced items such as cameras, perfume, and so on. Then, check the prices right here at home. You'll find, once you get to your destination, that the prices there are either higher than the ones at home or very little less, making it uneconomical to purchase it and carry it with you all the way through your trip. I've mentioned cameras and perfume, and to that list you can also add liquor in most countries. The allowable amount that you can bring in duty-free makes it less than worth while to carry glass bottles with you through planes, trains, and hotels.

I remember discovering, with delight and awe, a marvelous little place in Paris that sold my favorite liqueurs. It was in an alley and up three flights of stairs, and each time I was in Paris, I'd make my way there to sit at a small table and taste of the calvados and the cognacs. And each and every trip I'd end up carrying a neatly wrapped package of three or four prized bottles—until I discovered quite by accident that the charming Frenchman who owned the place also had a distributor in the United States not five blocks from my office and the price was but a dollar more!

So check the prices of everything you might buy—crystal, china, even imported clothing—since most manufacturing countries have an export line and a domestic line, the former one frequently of better quality than you can buy overseas at its source.

DUTY-FREE SHOPS

What I've suggested earlier also goes for the duty-free shops around the world, located at airports, aboard ships, in hotels, or at little shopping areas in the towns and cities. There was a time when those shops were literally a bonanza of bargains, but that time is long past in most places. I have found many of them to be much higher in price on many items, very little lower on others.

The fantasy, in many cases, overshadows the reality. Some cities have gotten their reputations as bargain capitals of the world—perfume in Paris, for example, or cameras in Hong Kong and Tokyo. The latter two places no longer deserve the accolades. Hong Kong has gotten terribly expensive and Tokyo is one of the most costly cities in the world—from hotels and food to cameras and other electronic equipment. The woolens in Australia, where they actually raise the sheep, are generally manufactured in Europe rather than at home, so the purchaser is also paying transportation costs both ways.

If you do decide to buy clothing overseas, keep in mind that the sizes are measured quite differently than they are at home. The accompanying chart may help you to work it out on the spot.

THE VALUE ADDED TAX

Some western European countries have levied what is called a *value added tax* (VAT) for purchases in their own shops. However, these taxes are only for the people who reside there and not for the tourist. In many instances, the VAT can run up to 17 percent of a purchase price, and it is refundable to you by merely following the proper procedures:

- When you make your purchase, fill out the proper forms right at the store.

- Get to the airport early on departure and *do not check* your luggage through until you have gone to the VAT counter to declare your purchase and hand in your form. There are times that the officials want to validate the purchase and to see that you are actually carrying it out of the country.

- A check for the amount of the VAT will be mailed to you at your home address.

I have one final word of advice about shopping, and you may accept it or refuse it as you wish. I remember one of the first overseas trips that I took, and all my friends telephoned with lists of the things they wanted me to find for them in Paris or Rome or Bangkok. Bit by bit, the list grew until it covered two full pages. Good naturedly, I thought that it would be fun to bring back all those simple little items for my friends. It taught me a lesson. Some things were not available, others required two or more trips to shops that were closed or out of stock. The time spent on shopping for friends soon became time away from museums, sight-seeing, and my own travel pleasure. With few exceptions,

MEN

_____ SUITS, SWEATERS AND OVERCOATS _____

American and British:	34	36	38	40	42	44	46	48
European:		44	46	48	50	52	54	56	58

_____ SHIRTS _____

American and British:	14	14½	15	15½	16	16½	17	17½
European:		36	37	38	39	40	41	42	43

_____ SOCKS _____

American and British:	9½	10	10½	11	11½	12	12½
European:	39	40	41	42	43	44	45

_____ SHOES _____

American:	7	7½	8	8½	9	9½	10	10½	11	11½
British:	6½	7	7½	8	8½	9	9½	10	10½	11
European:	39	40	41	42	43	43	44	44	45	45

_____ HATS _____

American:	6⅝	6¾	6⅞	7	7⅛	7¼	7⅜	7½	7⅝
British:	6½	6⅝	6¾	6⅞	7	7⅛	7¼	7⅜	7½
European:	53	54	55	56	57	58	59	60	61

GLOVE sizes are the same as in the U.S.A.

WOMEN

_____ DRESSES, SUITS AND COATS _____

American:	8	10	12	14	16	18
British:	30	32	34	36	38	40
European:	36	38	40	42	44	46

_____ BLOUSES AND SWEATERS _____

American:	32	34	36	38	40	42	44
British:	34	36	38	40	42	44	46
European:	40	42	44	46	48	50	52

___ DRESSES AND COATS (Children's and Junior Misses) ___

American:	2	4	6	8	10	13	15
British and European:	1	2	5	7	9	10	12

_____ STOCKINGS _____

American and British:	8	8½	9	9½	10	10½	11
European:	35	36	37	38	39	40	41

_____ SHOES _____

American:	5	5½	6	6½	7	7½	8	8½	9
British:	3½	4	4½	5	5½	6	6½	7	7½
European:	35	35	36	37	38	38	38½	39	40

GLOVE sizes are the same as in the U.S.A.

(All size equivalents are approximate)
American sizes apply in Canada and Mexico

I have simply made it a habit *not* to shop for friends who ask for special items. I think that you will find the same problems as you set off on your trip. Your time is limited—it is *your* vacation; you can simply graciously tell them that you just could not find the item overseas. For those of you who like to shop for friends, just ignore what I have written, and enjoy.

THE GREAT GAME OF CUSTOMS ROULETTE

I have heard the mutterings and whisperings on every trip that I've ever taken. Over the roar of the jet, someone says, "Are you going to declare it?" This is followed by a long discussion about the pros and cons of "getting it through" and, frankly, I don't know what the final decision is. If you understand the U.S. Customs rules and if you realize that a totally honest declaration will bring help from the Customs Agent in trying to achieve the lowest possible duty, and, if added to all that, you understand that these people have really seen it all, know what almost every package contains when it's carried by a returning vacationer, then it really doesn't pay. The penalties can be very severe—confiscation of the item for nondeclaration, plus a fine, plus a possible jail sentence if the item is valuable enough.

You probably overpaid for the article to begin with, just because you were a North American. Why, then, would you quibble about a small duty that is levied legitimately on some of the souvenirs that will always remind you of the trip? And everyone says, at this point, "Who me?" Well, maybe not you—but I sure have heard a lot of stories from people who managed to smuggle back a $20 item on which the duty might have run as much as a dollar and a quarter! It is more important that you understand just what it is that you can bring back home and just what items are not allowed into the United States for various reasons.

First of all, your duty-free allowance is currently $300 per person ($600 from the U.S. Virgin Islands, Guam, and American Samoa). Keep all your sales receipts when you make your purchases. And, if you decide to ask the local store owner to give you a receipt for less than the value of the item, also remember that Customs Agents are quite familiar with the current prices of almost anything you can think of.

• If you purchase clothing abroad, it is dutiable even if you then wear it and consider it "used."

278

- If you buy anything in a duty-free shop abroad, it is only duty-free where you bought it, not back in the United States.

- Some items from developing countries are now allowed into the United States duty-free.

- Any gift given to you abroad is also subject to duty.

- Many antiques are duty-free. They must be over 100 years old and you will have to show verification from the seller attesting to that fact.

IMPORTING PETS AND ANIMALS

If you are planning to import any unusual items, be sure you check with U.S. Customs before you leave home. For example, there are special restrictions for birds such as parakeets and parrots, turtles, and all kinds of pets. Monkeys may not be imported as pets, while your family dog will need full identification papers and a rabies certificate with date of vaccination and the signature of a licensed veterinarian. The rabies vaccination is not required for cats.

For further information about the restrictions and rules on importing animals, whether as pets or for other reasons, there are two booklets available. The first one has been recommended several times by me—*Health Information for International Travel,* and the other one is *How to Import Pets but Not Disease.* Both are available from: U.S. Public Health Service, Center for Disease Control, Atlanta, GA 30333.

On the other hand, if your questions are of a more general nature with regard to Customs regulations, write for this booklet: *Customs Hints for Returning U.S. Residents: Knowing Before You Go,* U.S. Customs Service, P.O. Box 7118, Washington, DC 20044.

WHAT YOU CANNOT BRING BACK

The most complicated area of all is the importation of food, plant, and animal products. If you are going to visit farm areas or, for some reason, you must bring home items that fit into those three categories, I'd suggest that you

279

send for: *Travelers' Tips on Bringing Food, Plant and Animal Products into the United States,* Superintendent of Documents, U.S. Government Printing Office, Washington, DC 20402.

In spite of what most people think, the personal luggage and carryon baggage of international travelers are major channels in the spread of agricultural pests and disease. The booklet is fascinating to glance through. It explains that you *can* import dried bamboo poles, necklaces made of seeds, coconuts without husks, canned fish, rocks and minerals, dried insects, or canned fruits. You *cannot* import the insides of the bamboo, necklaces made of jequirity beans, coconuts with husks, live insects, and many fresh fruits.

Hay, straw, and grass are prohibited. Dried herbs are not. Most nuts are admitted. Acorns are not. Sea shells can be collected and brought in, but snail shells must be empty and thoroughly cleaned. The answer is "yes" on most kinds of vegetables, but "no" on sweet potatoes and corn on the cob. It is, indeed, complicated, and it pays to check before you find that you have carried it with you in vain, just as the lovely woman who sat next to me on a trip home from Italy.

She was charming, she was radiant, she could have been my grandmother or the Italian grandmother of anyone on that plane. She sat next to me in the middle seat after we had boarded in Rome for the nonstop flight to the United States. On her lap she held a large tray covered with cloth and then wrapped in newspaper, and she kept it there throughout the entire trip. I had no idea what it was that she was guarding so intensely, no concept of what lay under that bulging wrapper.

One time during the trip, she asked to be excused to visit the lavatory in the rear of the plane, and she gave the huge platter to me to hold on my lap while she was gone. I could not peek—the paper was tied on tightly, but it was heavy. It was *very* heavy, and a marvelous aroma wafted up from the platter to my nose. She returned and I still had no better idea of what was in the bundle.

When we arrived in New York, I decided to follow her through to Customs. My curiosity was getting the better of me. Finally, we both arrived at the same line and I let her get in front of me so that I could watch. Tenderly, the Customs Officer unwrapped the package, and there, lying in all its glory, a gift to her family here in the United States, was *a huge roast suckling pig,* an apple stuffed in its mouth. The Customs Agent shook his head, then looked at me. It was a difficult moment. For, after all that time, with an entire trip behind her, the beautiful gift had to be *confiscated.* I shall never forget her face when it happened.

But then, I wondered—if I had known what it was when we were on the plane, would I have had the heart to tell her that it would be taken away when we reached New York? I realized, too, in that instant, that I was truly sorry that I had not known about the suckling pig. Think for a moment what might have happened—she could have given it up to me right on the plane, and 135 passengers might have feasted as no other airline passengers ever had. It would have been the most memorable picnic in the sky!

"HELLO AND GOODBYE"

... In Wistful Conclusion

Every travel book wishes its readers a "bon voyage" (or similar farewell in 27 languages). I shall not do so, for I know that your trip will be a good one and that somewhere on your way to the airport, the echo of everyone's good advice will still be ringing in your ears. Did-you-take-your-passport-your-foreign-currency-your-hotel-reservations-and-your-woolen-sweater-in-case-it-gets-cool-at-night-and-your-lightweight-suit-in-case-it-gets-too-warm-at-night-and-did-you-remember . . . .

Possibly you and I shall pass one another on the way, or sit next to one another on an airplane. Each of us will have been sleepless with excitement the night before, for it does not change even after so many years. For you—and for me—there is only one reason that any book like this is ever written—to make the trip easier and much more fun, to travel in good health and with comfort. It is the only way to go. And so, as your friends stand on the pier and in the airport and shout the echoing "Bon voyage," I can only wish you just one important word, and I hope that you carry it with you wherever you may eventually wander: *"Enjoy!"*

282

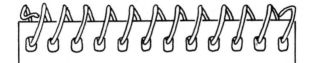

USE THESE PAGES
TO MAKE
THE GOING
EASIER

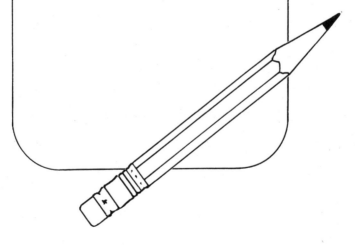

BEFORE YOU GO:

Make note of your passport number and date of issue, generic names of your drug prescriptions, emergency telephone numbers, names and addresses you might need at your destination.

ON THE TRIP:

Jot down currency conversion information, names of restaurants and shops you've discovered, names and addresses of new-found friends, plus other travel tips.

WHEN YOU RETURN:

Pass your tips on to your friends for their own forthcoming trips as well as to the author, c/o Rodale Press, 33 E. Minor Street, Emmaus, Pennsylvania 18049. Now that you've been patient enough to read all my stories, I'm ready to listen to yours.

INDEX